Treating Addicted Offenders in Community Settings (course) nance

Substance Abuse Treatment with Correctional Clients
Practical Implications for Institutional and Community Settings

Barbara Sims, PhD
Editor

D0217555

Routledge
Taylor & Francis Group
NEW YORK AND LONDON

First Published by

The Haworth Press, Inc., 10 Alice Street, Binghamton, NY 13904-1580.

This edition published 2011 by Routledge
711 Third Avenue, New York, NY 10017
2 Park Square, Milton Park, Abingdon, Oxon, OX14 4RN

Cover design by Marylouise E. Doyle.

Library of Congress Cataloging-in-Publication Data

Substance abuse treatment with correctional clients : practical implications for institutional and community settings / Barbara Sims, editor.
     p. cm.
   Includes bibliographical references and index.
   ISBN 0-7890-2126-9 (hard : alk. paper) — ISBN 0-7890-2127-7 (soft : alk. paper)
    1. Substance abuse—Treatment. 2. Prisoners—Drug use. 3. Prisoners—Mental health services.
4. Criminals—Rehabilitation. I. Sims, Barbara.

RC564.S83752 2004
365'.66—dc22

2004009808

Substance Abuse Treatment
with Correctional Clients
Practical Implications
for Institutional
and Community Settings

HAWORTH Criminal Justice, Forensic Behavioral Sciences, & Offender Rehabilitation
Nathanial J. Pallone, PhD
Senior Editor

To the criminal justice faculties at both
the University of Arkansas at Little Rock
and Sam Houston State University
who encouraged me and provided me
with excellent role models

CONTENTS

ABOUT THE EDITOR

Barbara Sims, PhD, is Faculty Director for the Center for Survey Research and Associate Professor of Criminal Justice at Penn State Harrisburg. Dr. Sims is the 2002 winner of the James A. Jordan, Jr. Teaching Award. She is Co-Principal Investigator of a grant with the Pennsylvania Commission on Crime and Delinquency, the focus of which is to evaluate police/probation partnership programming across Pennsylvania, and a second grant that provides research support services to the Project Safe Neighborhoods Task Force for the Middle District of Pennsylvania. Her interests include development and evaluation of criminological theory, public opinion research on crime and criminal justice, issues of punishment in the American criminal justice system, institutional- and community-based corrections, juvenile law and justice, and domestic violence.

Dr. Sims has been published in the *Journal of Contemporary Criminal Justice, Criminal Justice Policy Review, Corrections Compendium, Policing, The Police Quarterly,* and *Corrections Management Quarterly,* among others. She has also been published in *Americans View Crime and Justice: A National Survey of Public Opinion;* the *Handbook in Criminal Justice Administration;* the *Handbook of Clinical Sociology;* and the *Encyclopedia of Juvenile Justice.* She is Editor in Chief of *Critical Criminology: An International Journal* and is a manuscript reviewer for such publications as *Crime and Delinquency, Crime and Justice Review,* and the *Journal of Criminal Justice.* She serves on the Executive Board of the Academy of Justice Sciences as Region 1 Trustee. She is also a member of the American Society of Criminology, the Northeastern Association of Criminal Justice Sciences, the Pennsylvania Criminal Justice Educators Association, the American Association of University Women, and Pi Gamma Mu.

CONTRIBUTORS

Dawn Marie Baletka is a doctoral candidate in the College of Criminal Justice, Sam Houston State University.

Diane Baune is a substance abuse counselor with the Idaho Department of Corrections.

Georgia Calhoun, PhD, is an associate professor and coordinator of the Community Counseling Program in the Department of Counseling and Human Development Services at the University of Georgia.

Paul J. Cohen, MEd, is a doctoral candidate in the Department of Counseling and Human Development Services at the University of Georgia.

Debbie S. Cunningham, MSCJ, is pursuing doctoral studies in Spanish at the University of Texas, Austin.

Jed Dayley is a probation officer in Twin Falls, Idaho.

M. A. "Toni" DuPont-Morales is an associate professor of criminal justice in the School of Public Affairs, Penn State Harrisburg, where she directs the Capital College Honors Program.

Brian A. Glaser, PhD, is a professor and director of training in counseling psychology in the Department of Counseling and Human Development Services, College of Education, at the University of Georgia.

James W. Golden, PhD, is an associate professor of criminal justice in the Criminal Justice Program at the University of Arkansas at Little Rock.

Mark Gornik is the director of the Bureau of Offender Programs for the Idaho Department of Corrections.

Craig Hemmens, PhD, is an associate professor and chairperson, Department of Criminal Justice Administration, Boise State University, Idaho.

Cheryl Deluca Johnson, MEd, is on the staff of the Metro Atlanta Recovery Residences.

Kristin Kjaer is a research analyst in the Bureau of Offender Programs, Idaho Department of Corrections.

TK Logan, PhD, is an associate professor, Center on Drug and Alcohol Research, Department of Psychiatry, College of Medicine, University of Kentucky.

Cindy Noon is an assistant research analyst in the Bureau of Offender Programs, Idaho Department of Corrections.

Allan L. Patenaude, PhD, is an assistant professor of criminal justice, University of Arkansas at Little Rock.

Robert A. Shearer, PhD, is a professor of criminal justice, Sam Houston State University.

Tres Stefurak, MEd, is a doctoral candidate in the Department of Counseling and Human Development Services, University of Georgia.

Mary K. Stohr, PhD, is a professor, Department of Criminal Justice Administration, Boise State University.

William E. Stone, PhD, is a professor of criminal justice, Southwest Texas State University.

Robert Walker, MSW, LCSW, is an assistant professor, Center on Drug and Alcohol Research, Department of Psychiatry, College of Medicine, University of Kentucky.

Preface

This volume had its remote origins when, in conjunction with the task of developing reporting protocols for Pennsylvania's Restrictive Intermediate Punishment (RIP) program (further detailed in Chapter 9), I began to immerse myself in the research literature dealing specifically with the issues associated with treating the substance-addicted offender, in particular with studies that evaluated empirically reduction in not only substance use but also criminal offending following treatment. The chapters that constitute this volume grew from correspondence with scholars and practitioners around the country with strong expertise in those focal concerns. From correspondence with—and among and between—leading researchers and clinicians, the idea for this book germinated.

I thank the contributors for allowing me a wide range of discretion in "adjusting" their original work so that, collectively, they would more appropriately align one with the other. Without such a commitment, the work could not have moved forward.

The contributing authors and I express gratitude to the late Dr. N. J. Pallone of Rutgers University, senior editor of the Criminal Justice and Forensic Behavioral Science book series at The Haworth Press, and to The Haworth Press for assisting and guiding us toward a finished product that adequately addresses the needs of both clinical practitioners and academics.

Nor could I have completed this project without the support of several key individuals. The Pennsylvania Commission on Crime and Delinquency (PCCD) has supported my research and related activities, as has Penn State Harrisburg. Dr. Steve Peterson, director of the School of Public Affairs, provided me with wonderful research assistants across the life of this project, beginning with the early stages of the RIP project. Wenbo Shi will long be remembered for his contribution to this project, as will my current research assistant, Hui Meng. Most important, much appreciation is expressed to my husband, Lonnie Daniel, who never ceased to understand my need to sacrifice our leisure time to this project.

Although the works presented in this text provide a sound picture of the issues currently addressed in corrections treatment studies, there is, of course, much more to be discovered and disseminated to corrections administrators, managers, and program providers. We who have contributed here hope that this text will, at the very least, provide some basic information that policymakers, researchers, and clinicians can use and, at the same time, will pique in them an interest in searching for additional material that is constantly coming online.

Introduction

Barbara Sims

The 2001 National Household Survey on Drug Abuse revealed that there are about 2.8 million dependent drug users, with about 1.5 million individuals determined to be less severe users (Office of National Drug Control Policy [ONDCP], 2002). This annual self-report study of drug use includes questions operationalized using definitions for drug abuse from the *Diagnostic and Statistical Manual of Mental Disorders* (DSM-IV-TR). The DSM-IV defines drug dependence as positive responses to questions concerning difficulty in cutting down on use, drug tolerance, drug withdrawal symptoms, and experience with a host of mental and physical health problems. Drug abuse, although less severe, is still a critical problem for many and is characterized as experiencing a variety of social problems (work, family, school, etc.), engaging in risk-taking behavior, and being subjected to criminal sanctions associated with abuse (DUIs, for example) (ONDCP, 2002).

In their annual report titled "National Drug Control Strategy" (2002), the ONDCP reports that less than 1 million of the 4.3 million individuals found to be either drug dependent or drug abusing received treatment in the year prior to the 2001 household study. These figures align with an earlier 1994 estimate by Kessler et al. (1994) that only 8 percent of the general population which reported some problems with drugs or alcohol in their lifetimes (27 percent of the general population) had received treatment.

A 1988 study revealed some dramatic changes over time (since the 1960s) in alcohol consumption in American society (Hilton, 1988). This is especially true for young (between the ages of twenty-one and thirty-four), white males. Over time, this particular population has engaged more and more in episodes of heavy drinking (eight or more drinks per day). Hilton (1988) was able to tease out this finding from examining a series of self-report studies from 1964 through 1984 that seemed to indicate stability across these years for both males and females when it comes to the frequency of alcohol use and the quantity of alcohol consumed per incident. Similarly, Hasin, Grant, & Harford (1990) found a rise in the prevalence of alcohol-related problems occurring among male drinkers in the twenty-two to fifty-nine age group. Considering alcohol abuse and alcohol dependence together, Grant et al. (1991), in a longitudinal study using the DSM-IV criteria for defining abuse and dependence, found that roughly 13.76 million Americans could be described as either one or both of these types of alcohol users.

In 1997, through the Survey of Inmates in State and Federal Correctional Facilities, 51 percent of federal and state prisoners reported being under the influence of drugs and/or alcohol while committing their present offense, and about 33 percent of state and 25 percent of federal inmates reported receiving treatment for substance addiction since they had been admitted to prison (Mumola, 1999). Although there seemed to be little variation by offense type for state prisoners regarding being under the influence at the time of the incident, for federal inmates, violent offenders were more likely to have been using drugs and/or alcohol at the time of their offense (40 percent) than were offenders charged with other crimes (Mumola, 1999).

Of the 22 percent of federal inmates who reported using drugs at the time of the offense, 11 percent were more likely to report the type of drug as marijuana, 9 percent as cocaine/crack, 3 percent as heroin/opiates, with the remainder of inmates reporting the drug to be depressants, stimulants, hallucinogens, or inhalants (Mumola, 1999). Slightly more state inmates reported using drugs at the time of their current offense (33 percent), with 15 percent reporting that drug to be marijuana, 15 percent cocaine/crack, 6 percent heroin/opiates, and rest the same as those drugs previously mentioned for federal inmates (Mumola, 1999).

Reported drug use in the month prior to the current offense varied by type of inmate as well. Whereas 45 percent of federal inmates reported usage for any drug in the month leading up to the current arrest, 57 percent of state inmates did so. These differences hold up when it comes to the abuse of alcohol. Although both state and federal inmates were as likely to experience problems with alcohol as with drugs, a higher number of state inmates than federal inmates reported having engaged in risky behaviors, such as driving while under the influence, domestic disputes, or physical fighting (Mumola, 1999). Mumola (1999:8), after his review of the data from the survey, concluded that "three-quarters of all prisoners can be characterized as alcohol- or drug-involved offenders."

Even in light of evidence indicating the critical nature of substance abuse by correctional clients, data from the Bureau of Justice Statistics estimate that about 150,000 state inmates are released from prison each year without having undergone any type of treatment for their addiction (ONDCP, 2002). The present Bush administration, however, has committed funds to the states to assist in the implementation of treatment programs in prison through the Residential Substance Abuse Treatment program, and in the federal system, funds have been designated for drug treatment, with a goal of reaching 100 percent participation in these programs, with funding for treatment following the inmate into the community once he or she has been released (ONDCP, 2002).

The overall focus of this book is treating the substance-addicted correctional client. The problems associated with abusing drugs and/or alcohol are sometimes criminal in nature. Although no straight line can be drawn between drug use and crime, enough evidence is available to suggest that a relationship exists between these two social phenomena. The debate about the strength and direction of that relationship is ongoing and is the subject for another day. Suffice it to say here that the evidence is clear about the number of correctional clients who enter the criminal justice system reporting having used, as described previously, just prior to their arrest and who report problems in this area.

Nor does this book tackle the important issue embedded in the question, "Just how good are our measures of drug/alcohol abuse and/or dependence?" I certainly recognize the problems in this area. Exactly at what point does an individual cross the line between "use" and "abuse"? How wide or narrow is the line between "dependency" and "abuse"? These are important questions, but again, the subject for another text. Although they may be touched on briefly in the following chapters, the important issue here is the fact that many correctional clients admit that their use of drugs and/or alcohol has caused a host of problems for themselves, and more often than not, for others as well.

In the following chapters, the terminology may change somewhat. In some chapters, the author(s) may use the terms *substance abuse, drug abuse, alcohol abuse,* or *drug and/or alcohol abuse* to define an individual dependent variable. No attempt has been made here to standardize the definition of someone who abuses substances: alcohol, drugs, or alcohol and drugs. Also, it is noted that alcohol is indeed a drug, but perhaps because it is legal, whereas other drugs are not, it is sometimes separated into a different category. Differences in terminology were allowed, and each chapter is a stand-alone treatment of the subject matter.

This text is divided into three major parts. Part I lays the foundation for the subsequent chapters through a review of such topics as theoretical explanations for substance abuse, "best practice" treatment programs for substance abusers, issues associated with substance abuse in the corrections environment, and the debate that is ongoing over the use of coerced or mandated treatment. Part II includes chapters that address treating the substance-addicted offender in the institutional setting, and Part III includes works that describe community-based treatment programs and some of the problems associated with them. The text closes, in Part IV, with a description of correctional-based substance abuse treatment programs for both juveniles and females. Taken as a whole, these works are replete with recommendations by the authors for corrections administrators and treatment providers alike.

As an aid to the reader, I have included several discussion questions at the end of each chapter. These questions are meant to guide readers through the process of thinking critically about some of the major policy issues faced by those who provide substance abuse treatment under what can only be described as coercive circumstances.

The issue of treating substance-addicted individuals is one that has found its way, in the most recent past, to the top of a priority list in local communities. This means that the stigma sometimes associated with this particular group of individuals has begun to wane somewhat. It could be that we have come to realize, as has been pointed out by the medical community, that addiction is a disease, and because it is, it deserves specialized treatment no less so than does any other disease. Leshner (1998:3) defines addiction as a "chronic, relapsing illness, characterized by compulsive drug seeking and use." He points out that

Many, perhaps most, people see drug abuse and addiction as social problems, to be handled only with social solutions, particularly through the criminal justice system. On the other hand, science has taught that drug abuse and addiction are as much health problems as they are social problems. The consequence of this perception gap is a significant delay in gaining control over the drug abuse problem. (Leshner, 1998:3)

Perhaps the perception gap is closing, at least to a certain extent. Much of the information presented in the subsequent chapters suggests that it is, at the very least, growing narrower. With much more attention now being given to treating individuals who have come in contact with the criminal justice system, and who have been found to be addicted to substances, we might say that we have come to recognize, as Leshner points out, that addiction is much more than a mere social problem that can be handled through the threat of criminal sanctions.

REFERENCES

Grant, D.F., Harford, T.C., Chou, P., Pickering, R., Dawson, D.A., Stinson, F.A., & Noble, J. (1991). Prevalence of DSM-III-R alcohol abuse and dependence. *United States, Alcohol Health and Research World, 15,* 91-96.

Hasin, D., Grant, B., & Harford, T. (1990). Male and female difference in liver cirrhosis mortality in the United States, 1961-1985. *Journal of Studies on Alcohol, 51,* 123-129.

Hilton, M.E. (1988). Trends in U.S. drinking patterns: Further evidence from the past 20 years. *British Journal of Addiction, 83* (3), 269-278.

Kessler, R.C., McGonagle, K.A., Zhao, S., Nelson, C.B., Eshelman, S., Wittchen, H.U., & Kandler, K.S. (1994). Lifetime and 12-month prevalence of DSM-III-R psychiatric disorders in the United States. *Archives of General Psychiatry, 51,* 8-19.

Leshner, A.I. (1998, October). Addiction is a brain disease and it matters. *National Institute of Justice Journal, 237,* 2-6.

Mumola, C.J. (1999). *Substance abuse and treatment, state and federal prisoners, 1997.* Washington, DC: Bureau of Justice Statistics.

Office of National Drug Control Policy. (2002). *National drug control strategy.* Washington, DC: U.S. Government Printing Office.

PART I:
THE NATURE OF THE PROBLEM

Myriad explanations exist for why people abuse substances. Among theorists and practitioners from major disciplines of study, a consensus has been reached about the multicausal nature of abuse. That is to say, the abuse of substances probably has many causes, not just one. Through an examination of studies that seek to cull out the major predictors of substance abuse, Chapter 1 by Sims lays the foundation for the chapters that follow. She does so by first discussing the major theoretical explanations for substance abuse, which she then follows up with a review of the major types of programs currently being used to treat the substance-addicted individual. She concludes Chapter 1 with a brief description of critical issues faced by correctional managers who attempt to implement "free-world" substance abuse programming in the prison and community-based correctional setting.

Chapter 2 by Golden and Sims examines further some of the issues of corrections-based substance abuse programming. This chapter deals specifically with those factors that have been found to be predictors of success and/or failure in these types of programs. They suggest, as do many of the authors in subsequent chapters, that unless these predictors are addressed, complete with the realization that clients will more than likely present with co-occurring problems, that treatment failures will be greater in number than treatment successes.

In Chapter 3, Shearer tackles the controversial issue of coerced treatment. He does so by laying out the arguments for and against coerced treatment in the correctional environment, using the concept of "motivation" and its many derivatives. It is, as Shearer argues, individual motivation for breaking the cycle of substance abuse that is the key turning point for this type of programming.

Chapter 1

Treating the Substance-Addicted Offender: Theory and Practice

Barbara Sims

The purpose of this chapter is to provide a foundation for the subsequent chapters. It does so through a look at well-known theoretical explanations for alcohol and drug abuse, followed by a review of the literature on treatment programs.

THEORETICAL EXPLANATIONS FOR ALCOHOL AND DRUG ABUSE

The theoretical explanations for alcohol and drug abuse are varied, and it is clear that one theory does not fit all individuals. Some use is connected to pleasure-seeking behavior, and the opportunity for the feelings associated with use seems worth the risks of encountering negative consequences (Jung, 2001). As Jung (2001) points out, some individuals become addicted as they increasingly come to rely on drugs or alcohol in their daily living. The major theories associated with the crossover of drug *use* to drug *addiction* include biological theory, psychological theory, developmental theory, and problem behavior theory. These theories are not to be viewed as holding adversarial positions; rather, they complement one another and produce a more complete picture of drug addiction when the overlap between them is taken into account.

Biological Theory

According to research by Tarter, Alterman, and Edwards (1985), biological characteristics may predispose individuals to problems with drug/alcohol use. Primarily, Tarter et al. (1985) found this to be the case in a study of adult males. Certain temperamental characteristics appeared to account for a higher risk of abusing alcohol, especially in males who began using alcohol at an early age. The researchers propose that alcohol may actually be more reinforcing in some individuals with a certain level of inherent sensitivity toward alcohol such that continued use, and eventual abuse, is the outcome (Tarter et al., 1985).

Sher's (1991) vulnerability model proposes a similar scenario as that of Tarter et al. (1985). In this model, innate dispositions of greater sensitivity to drugs seem to produce a greater reliance on drugs and alcohol as a method of relieving stress. This was particularly true of individuals who had not developed adequate coping skills (Sher, 1991). Similarly, the negative effect model suggests that drugs and alcohol are often used as a form of self-medication in individuals suffering from depression or recovering from some catastrophic life event (Jung, 2001).

When it comes to distinguishing one type of drug user from another, that is to say, in trying to determine which drugs are more likely to be involved in addiction and in what type of individual, much of the research suggests that types of individuals do not vary by much. Tarter, Moss, Arria, Mezzich, and Vanyukov (1992) argue that although the properties associated with the effects of drugs on individual neurology may differ and may determine the rate at which addiction occurs, drug-/alcohol-dependent individuals do not differ that much one from the other. At least, they do not differ in any neurophysiological sense. Rather, explanations for drug choice are more likely to be found in cultural or social norms, or related to the current laws associated with drug and alcohol use (Jung, 2001).

This is consistent with findings in the literature that associate addiction with lower levels of certain brain chemistries (dopamine, serotonin, etc.). According to Blum et al. (1995), most psychoactive drugs affect the levels of these chemicals in the brain by way of a series of neurotransmitters. In their study, for example, the administering of amino acid precursors to a group of alcohol-dependent individuals produced higher levels of dopamine and serotonin, which, in turn, reduced the craving for alcohol.

Psychological Theory

Much of individual knowledge about the use of drugs or alcohol takes place in the social setting. Social learning theory suggests that we learn drug use just as we learn any other type of behavior, through observing use by others (Bandura, 1977). This knowledge of what types of drugs are used, which are more socially accepted than others, and the effects of different types of drugs on individuals is easily acquired in a culture whose social norms tolerate certain levels of usage. As Jung (2001:167) says, "We acquire much knowledge about the effects of alcohol and other drugs before we actually use a specific drug."

Social learning theory also predicts drug abuse through individual self-efficacy, the degree to which self-esteem and self-confidence allow individuals to believe in their ability to cope with tasks and control outcomes (Jung, 2001). Individuals with a low sense of self-efficacy may turn to drugs and alcohol, as mentioned previously, to assist with stress reduction or to alleviate the discomfort associated with the introduction of noxious stimuli into one's life. This can be viewed as the "I give up" syndrome in individuals who are not confident in their ability to approach problems in a manner such that a positive outcome can be achieved.

An unfortunate outcome for people with low levels of self-efficacy, and thus a poorly developed set of coping skills, is that they will eventually alienate themselves from individuals who are not similarly situated. Learning theory predicts that the result of this alienation, the "hanging out with" other people who are themselves using and abusing drugs and alcohol, only reinforces this type of escapist behavior. This "reciprocal influence exists among members of this group" (Jung, 2001:168).

The Developmental Perspective

A great deal of overlap can be seen between social learning theory and many of the models for drug addiction found in the developmental perspective. This perspective argues from the standpoint that what we learn about drug and alcohol use as we develop provides the foundation for the more proximate precursors of use in adolescence and into adulthood (Jung, 2001).

In addition to this learning process or the modeling of behavior we see in others, Hawkins and Weis (1985) suggest that weak bonds to the key institutions of society, e.g., families and schools, can contribute to drug or alcohol dependency. So too could the lack of conventional role models in a young person's life. A chaotic home life with consistent parental arguing, for example, where arguing escalates to physical confrontations in front of the child can result in several negative outcomes for the child. Academic failure is one, and the other is the inability to develop the sort of interpersonal skills that individuals need in order to cope with life stressors, those skills important to the self-efficacy model discussed earlier (Jung, 2001).

This family interaction model is of major concern to Brook, Brook, Gordon, Whiteman, and Cohen (1990) who propose that adolescents with secure ties to affectionate parents and who have learned within the family more conventional values are less likely to experiment with drugs or alcohol and to hang out with kids who do. For example, the positive effects of maternal interest in the child cannot be overemphasized, according to Brook et al. (1990), when it comes to any deviant activity, including drug or alcohol use.

Problem Behavior Theory

In this final category of theoretical explanations for addiction (which by no means exhausts the literature surrounding this extremely complicated phenomenon) there is again a fair amount of overlap with those theories previously discussed. This area of thought covers

1. excuse theory;
2. self-handicapping theory;
3. self-awareness reduction theory;
4. tension reduction theory; and
5. stress response dampening theory.

Excuse theory, simply put, allows individuals to place blame for certain behavior on their drug or alcohol use. According to MacAndrew and Edgerton (1969), being under the influence of some substance is, in some circles, a socially accepted excuse for inappropriate behavior. "I was drinking" is often the lamentation of perpetrators of domestic violence, promising to stop drinking and thus the abusing behavior. Unfortunately, many victims of domestic violence also often blame their abuse on the drinking or drug-using behaviors of their perpetrators. Both parties engage in excusing such conduct because of the influence of drugs or alcohol.

In a similar vein, self-handicapping theory suggests that an overindulgence in drugs or alcohol often occurs prior to certain situations in which one believes that he or she is likely to fail (Jung, 2001). Lack of adequate social skills and the social learning theory again come into play. Learned expectations of "I am likely to fail because I have before in this type of situation" set individuals up for failure. Or, a past success can put pressure on individuals to keep performing at a certain level. Self-handicapping occurs when individuals believe that the past success must have been an anomaly given the past history of the individual. Indulging in drugs and/or alcohol prior to the upcoming event allows the individual to excuse the expected failure because of being under the influence.

J. Hull (1987) proposed that drugs and alcohol actually impair thinking processes, which can bring about a reduction in self-awareness, primarily the reality of the immediate moment. This, again, gives people under the influence of drugs or alcohol yet another excuse for having engaged in inappropriate or offensive behavior. "I wasn't aware of what I was doing, so I am not to blame" is often the expression used in these types of situations.

Both tension reduction theory and stress response dampening theory have been alluded to previously, and C. Hull's (1943) early research supports both. According to Hull (1943), any response that reduces discomfort will be sought out again when people are confronted with similar situations that produced the discomfort and the subsequent behavior that reduced it. Unfortunately, drug and alcohol use reduce tension or stress only temporarily. The pleasure of escaping some unpleasant situation is short-lived. Excessive use of drugs or alcohol actually *increases* tension and stress. The individual will, sooner or later, have to face up to the consequences, and in many cases to family members and friends. In other cases, individuals may be faced with criminal sanctions. For individuals who use substances as a means of relieving stress, the unlearning of this response is critical. Treatment approaches should include the introduction, or the learning of, alternative means of reducing or dealing with stress (Jung, 2001).

In short, the literature suggests that drug and alcohol abuse is multifaceted in nature and that there is no one single cause. Reasons for abusing drugs or alcohol vary from one individual to another depending on the biological disposition of that individual and a host of social, cultural, and psychological factors which most certainly vary from one person to another. If it is true that no one theory can explain substance abuse, it follows that there can be no "one size fits all" treatment program for this particular population.

TREATING SUBSTANCE ADDICTION

Just as the theoretical explanations for drug and/or alcohol abuse and dependence should be viewed together as a whole because of the overlap between and among them, so too should the programs that have been developed to combat abuse and dependence. Programs identified and discussed here are grounded in three basic categories: (1) pharmacological treatment programs, (2) psychotherapeutic programs, and (3) behavioral modification programs.

Pharmacological Treatment Programs

Administering drugs to alcohol- or drug-dependent individuals is usually a first step taken to alleviate the adverse effects of abstinence. During detoxification, some patients are, for example, administered such drugs as Librium or Valium to relieve the symptoms of anxiety and depression (Jung, 2001). Sometimes, however, drugs are administered to purposefully cause severe physical discomfort in the presence of other drugs. For alcoholics, disulfiram is often administered to block the elimination from the liver of toxins associated with drinking alcohol. Drinking while taking this drug causes extreme nausea and vomiting in the drinker (Brewer, 1993). Also, other drugs, such as naltrexone, have been found to block the effects of alcohol and thus reduce cravings and relapses (Volpicelli, Clay, Watson, & Volpicelli, 1995).

Other treatment programs, sometimes referred to as drug-replacement approaches, include a pharmacological approach as one component of treatment. Methadone maintenance programs are good examples of this approach.

Methadone Maintenance Treatment

Opiod addiction, in recent years, has become a major problem in the drug-treatment community. Data from the Office of National Drug Control Policy indicate there were almost 1 million heroin-dependent individuals in the United States and about 100,000 first-time users at the beginning of the twenty-first century (National Drug Court Institute [NDCI], 2002). In addition, data from the 1998 Monitoring the Future study reveal some use of heroin among the nation's high school students (1.4 percent of tenth graders) (NDCI, 2002).

One of the most widely known and studied treatment programs for heroin addiction is methadone maintenance (NDCI, 2002). For over three decades, methadone has been used in conjunction with other services to the client, e.g., counseling and medical attention. In most treatment programs, daily doses are administered by a registered nurse, with fewer doses given as the person becomes stable. Doses vary, not unlike any other drug, from one patient to another depending on need. Methadone is taken orally and is quickly absorbed into body tissue and released into the bloodstream. In most treatment programs, patients are tested regularly for the presence of both methadone and illegal drugs (NDCI, 2002). According to research conducted by several agencies (National Institute on Drug Abuse and the National Institute on Alcohol Abuse and Alcoholism), methadone treatment programs are highly effective in reducing the craving for heroin (NDCI, 2002).

Criticism for methadone treatment programs can be separated into two major areas. Some critics insist that it is nothing more than a drug substitution program, and others suggest that because a drug is still being ingested by addicted individuals, it does not reflect a true recovery program (NDCI, 2002). According to research, however, and as reported by the NDCI (2002), both arguments fall short. First, methadone does not cause euphoric effects in the patient as does heroin; it is taken orally as opposed to being administered through injection, snorting, or smoking, and it is released into the body over a course of time, giving it a duration of action much longer than that of heroin (twenty-four hours versus four hours). Second, much of the research points to the conclusion that the chemistry of the brain in heroin-addicted individuals may never return to its original state in heavy users, with about 80 percent of them relapsing within the first twelve months of the withdrawal of methadone treatment (NDCI, 2002). This finding supports the notion that methadone-treated offenders are indeed in a state of recovery while in treatment since use of heroin is drastically reduced during this phase of treatment.

The NDCI (2002:2) states that it has been "repeatedly demonstrated that 80% of the patients will reduce or eliminate crime as they remain in methadone treatment programs." Information from the NDCI (2002) also indicates that the economic benefits to taxpayers of treatment is somewhere in the area of a ratio of 4:1, with a four-dollar savings to taxpayers for every dollar spent on methadone treatment, with an average cost of 5,000 dollars per patient per year. It should be pointed out that this amount includes not only the drugs and the cost of administering them but also the costs associated with other services (counseling and medical care) that are provided in the clinical setting (NDCI, 2002).

Most methadone treatment programs are in the community and thus are used for the community-based correctional client. With, however, much of the research pointing to this treatment as an effective means of reducing recidivism, treatment providers and researchers are calling for the establishment of methadone treatment programs within the institutional setting. According to the NDCI (2002), to date, only Rikers Island in New York provides this type of treatment to heroin-addicted offenders. With 3,985 inmates treated in 2000, the program demonstrated a significant decrease in recidivism, with 76 percent of inmates continuing their care in the community upon release as part of their parole requirements (NDCI, 2002).

One final note about methadone maintenance treatment is called for. Addiction to heroin is considered a chronic condition, and as such, great care should be given to the treatment of these individuals.

> Just as psychiatrists are not expected to withdraw depressed patients from their antidepressant medications and, as physicians do not withdraw their patients from cardiovascular or other life sustaining medications that stabilize the patient and enable him/her to lead a normal life without struggling through the debilitating effects of an illness, methadone patients should not be

required to withdraw from a medication that improves their quality of life. (NDCI, 2002:4)

Psychotherapeutic Approaches

According to Jung (2001), psychotherapeutic approaches to the treatment of drug- or alcohol-dependent individuals emphasize communication between the individual and his or her therapist. This interaction often takes place in both the individual and the group setting. Through communication, the therapist hopes to identify in the patient background characteristics from early childhood as well as stressors and motivators in the individual's current life situation that might serve as precursors to alcohol or drug use (Jung, 2001). Through psychoanalysis, for example, the patient is taken through a series of steps designed to "break down client defenses, provide insight, and facilitate recovery" (Jung, 2001:425).

Greenson (1967) suggests that, through psychoanalysis, the patient and the therapist form a working alliance that helps break down the patient's resistance to treatment and change. It is hoped that the discovery of sometimes unconscious and underlying conflicts within the individual will allow for the development of changes not only in how the individual thinks about usage but also in usage behavior itself (Greenson, 1967).

Evaluations of the psychotherapeutic approach are hard to come by, particularly because most therapists rely primarily on years of experience with patients, many of whom have gone on to live drug-free lives. The problem, however, is that therapists sometimes attribute success to the *treatment,* not taking into account other intervening factors that might have been associated with that success (Jung, 2001). Too, and as pointed out by Jung (2001), many therapists do not want their programs evaluated and refuse to be part of any comprehensive program evaluation.

Further complicating the matter is the ethical dilemma of denying treatment to a control group. Patients would need to be randomly assigned to treatment if a true experimental design were to be undertaken. The control group is important if one wishes to establish causality, i.e., to be able to say, all things being equal, it was indeed the intervening treatment that brought about a change in the individual's behavior. The "all things being equal" expression refers to the fact that if both groups, those receiving the treatment and those not receiving the treatment, are randomly assigned, they probably will look very similar to each other. In other words, they are likely to exhibit similar sociodemographic characteristics (age, gender, race/ethnicity, level of education, income, etc.) as well as demonstrate similar motivational drives, or lack thereof, to seek treatment. Whereas therapists are reluctant to participate in the random assignment of treatment, researchers demand it if we are ever to establish the efficacy of the psychotherapeutic approach to treating the drug- or alcohol-addicted individual.

Rational Emotive Therapy

One psychotherapeutic model of treatment takes a somewhat different approach from the more typical one of examining the past for problems that might be associated with present behavior. Rational emotive therapy (RET) gets the patient to focus more on the present and on the future motivations for drug use. Ellis, McInerney, DiGuiseppe, and Yeager (1988) argue that psychological problems are based in irrational beliefs and that the solution, then, is to redirect patients' misplaced misconceptions about addiction. The role of the therapist who treats an alcoholic, for example, in RET is to continually challenge the facts of what the individual is saying. Quite often, alcoholics will use such statements as, "I am not an alcoholic because I don't drink every day," or "I need alcohol in order to relieve the tension associated with my job (or family, or school, etc.)." The therapist presents evidence to the contrary, forcing the alcoholic to realize the irrationality of what he or she is saying (Ellis et al., 1988).

Behavioral Modification Programs

Much of the literature regarding behavioral modification programs points out that these programs are very much grounded in learning theory and the concept of operant conditioning. Just as one learns to abuse substances by modeling the behavior of others, substance abusers can learn the positive social consequences of reducing substance abuse through observing the reactions from significant others to this change in behavior. As Jung (2001:428) points out, "Drug use is similar to any other behavior in the sense that it can be reinforced by the consequences of that behavior."

Contingency contracting is one such technique sometimes used by therapists. The client, for example, might enter into an arrangement with the therapist to deposit some sum of money that will be returned to the client if he or she completes the prescribed program of treatment (Pomerleau, Pertschuck, Adkins, & Brady, 1978). Or the client learns that continuing employment, as another example, is a positive outcome of regulating substance abuse. Positive reinforcement through the strengthening of ties to family and close friends is yet another example of the contingency agreement approach to treatment.

In a similar vein, *motivational enhancement training* approaches treatment by having the client assume the responsibility for wanting to make changes. This approach is much more proactive on the part of clients because it requires them to think about how they would like their lives to be, and to see the discrepancies between those goals and their current situations (Miller, 1995). It is hoped that through this process, clients will develop lacking self-efficacy skills and a belief that "they can influence outcomes" (Jung, 2001:429).

Other Treatment Issues

In addition to the importance of recognizing the reasons associated with substance abuse and for developing a better understanding of the various approaches to changing such abuse, it is equally important to attend to such issues as screening procedures, matching individuals to the type of treatment that will work best for them, and the role that motivation plays in the recovery process.

One of the major goals of treatment has been to develop methods for detecting problems early on as a means to closing the door to future and more severe problems (Jung, 2001). Developed by Selzer in the 1970s (see Selzer, 1971), the Michigan Alcohol Screening Test (MAST) uses a series of questions that addresses the individual's perceptions of his or her drinking habits, perceptions of friends and/or relatives, and any negative consequences associated with drinking patterns or habits. Storgaard, Neilsen, and Gluud (1994) conducted an evaluation of validity studies of the MAST, discovering mixed and inconclusive results. One of the problems with this method of diagnosing substance-abusing behavior is, of course, related to honest reporting by individuals. It could be that MAST-type diagnostic techniques could work for those already in treatment, assuming that this population has accepted the fact that they have a problem, but using them for individuals who are not yet in treatment could prove problematic (Jung, 2001). Much work is needed in the area of early screening for individuals who are becoming, or already are, abusers of drugs and/or alcohol.

As critical as early screening is to identifying problems with substance abuse, assigning individuals to treatment programs once abuse has been established is, arguably, even more critical. As seen in the review of the literature on theory and practice, an approach that does not take into consideration each individual's reasons for substance-abusing behavior, and just assumes that what works for one individual will work for another, will completely miss the mark. In many situations, a mixed-modality approach may be called for, and this is where screening techniques are especially important.

Research by Babor, Kranzler, and Lauerman (1989) found that matching alcoholics to programs was more successful when a variety of screening tools were used. These tools included a physical exam, blood work, diagnostic interviews, personality tests, and two self-report inventories. The researchers discovered significant differences between males and females when it comes to the type of program that might work best. For example, the self-report measures were more successful at differentiating among males but less successful for identifying high-risk females (Babor et al., 1989). Further, Cooney, Kadden, Litt, and Getter (1991) found that mismatched patients were less successful than were matched patients, and over a two-year period.

Given the picture of substance abusers as possessing low self-esteem and not being equipped with positive coping skills, it is not surprising that many do not have the necessary motivation to refrain from using substances when undergoing treatment. In fact, and as pointed out by Jung (2001:453), "When treatment fails, it is often attributed to the client's lack of motivation, not to the lack of therapist skill or to the inappropriateness of the treatment." Measuring motivation, however, is somewhat problematic and is more often assumed to either be present, as is the case when one successfully completes a program, or absent, when clients fail to complete a program and relapse. Ryan, Plant, and O'Malley (1995) suggest that patients who show some evidence of a high internal motivation to succeed, coupled with high external motivations (expectations and support from family, friends, or even the therapist himself or herself), are more likely to succeed. The highest risk for failure to succeed, not surprisingly, is the absence of internalized motivation even in the presence of strong external motivations.

IMPLICATIONS FOR THE CORRECTIONAL ENVIRONMENT

The theories and treatment programs associated with substance-addicted individuals, and the subsequent research, reveal that a great deal of work has gone into this particular area of study. The literature reviewed here spans six decades, and the treatment community now has reliable evidence on which to base approaches to treating this social problem. Beyond the scope of this work are such issues as the availability of treatment in some communities and the costs of treatment to the clients. Data suggest, as reported in the Introduction, that only 8 percent of the general population who self-describe themselves as having a problem with drugs and/or alcohol report receiving treatment for that problem. It is not reaching, then, to assume that lack of availability of treatment programs in local communities, coupled with the sometimes high and out-of-reach costs of substance abuse treatment, might be correlated with the high number of individuals who are not being treated.

As difficult as it might be for substance-addicted individuals in the "free world" to obtain the treatment needed to assist them in refraining from abusing drugs and/or alcohol, the problem is exacerbated in the correctional setting. Data also show, as reported in the preceding section, that a majority of both state and federal inmates report that they have not received treatment for their substance abuse problems while incarcerated. With corrections administrators faced with making critical decisions about where to allocate scarce resources, sometimes substance abuse treatment programs, just like any other type of prison program, are forced to take a backseat to other budget areas such as security and daily care of the inmate population.

The Federal Bureau of Prisons, however, has sought to meet its legislated-mandated goal of ensuring that all *eligible* inmates receive some type of drug treatment prior to their release (Office of National Drug Control Policy [ONDCP], 2001). As reported in Table 1.1, the majority of federal inmates are treated in residential and drug education programs, with the remainder treated in transitional and nonresi-

TABLE 1.1. Inmates in Federal Bureau of Prisons treatment programs—1998

Program type	Number of inmates
Residential	10,006
Transitional	6,591
Nonresidential	5,038
Drug education	12,992
Total	34,627

Source: Federal Bureau of Prisons, 1999.

dential settings, with nearly 35,000 inmates treated in these programs in 1998 (ONDCP, 2001). The ONDCP (2001) estimates that the price tag for this treatment is approximately $2,941 (using 1993 and 1995 figures) per episode and that treatment results in an average treatment benefit per client of $9,177.

At the state level, many states have received funds from federal block grants for Residential Substance Abuse Treatment (RSAT) as part of the 1994 Violent Crime Control and Law Enforcement Act. This act calls for states receiving funding to rely on findings from the scientific literature to guide them in the development and implementation of treatment programs. An evaluation of Maryland's RSAT program revealed several interesting factors, many of which align with the literature on theory and practice (Taxman, Silverman, & Bouffard, 2000). First is the recognition that it is important to match a person's stage of change (i.e., the extent to which the client recognizes that he or she has a problem and is motivated to make changes in his or her behavior) to type of treatment modality. Second, the major components of the program emphasize developing cognitive and social skills and increasing individuals' self-efficacy. Further, the RSAT program encourages individuals to participate in peer groups in order to "heighten individual awareness of specific attitudes or behavioral patterns to be modified" (Taxman et al., 2000:iv).

The Maryland RSAT program, and other institutional-based programs, closely follow recommendations from Rawson, Obert, McCann, and Varinelli-Casey (1993) that call for correctional managers to implement programs grounded firmly in seven important areas from a cognitive-behavioral framework:

1. Implementing a psychoeducational component (awareness of the problem and the negative consequences of substance-abusing behaviors)
2. Identifying high-risk situations for relapse and the warning signs of relapse
3. Developing appropriate coping skills
4. Developing new, prosocial lifestyle behaviors
5. Increasing self-efficacy
6. Dealing with relapse when it occurs
7. Monitoring closely drug and/or alcohol use

Further, and as suggested by Prochaska, DiClemente, and Norcross (1992), there is a need for correctional treatment providers and criminal justice personnel to recognize that recovery from substance abuse is not perfectly linear. In fact, recovery often involves individuals vacillating between various stages of acceptance of their problem. These stages range from the precontemplation stage, in which the individual does not recognize that a problem exists, to the action stage in which the individual begins to devote a great deal of time and energy into making behavioral changes, to the final maintenance stage where work begins on avoiding episodes of relapse (Prochaska et al., 1992). In institutional- or community-based corrections, and more often than not, the realization that recovery from substance abuse is a step-up/step-down/step-up process is critical yet is difficult to accept given the requirements of institutional rules or probation/parole conditions of supervision.

Much of the literature on treating the substance-addicted correctional client addresses predictors of success or failure in the correctional environment. Some of these issues are addressed in the next chapter and, at least in part, in the subsequent chapters.

DISCUSSION QUESTIONS

1. Discuss the role that cultural norms associated with drug and/or alcohol use play when it comes to substance abuse or addiction.

2. Much of the literature suggests that substance abuse occurs when individuals have a biological predisposition to abuse drugs and/or alcohol and, at the same time, when they observe around them the use of these substances by others. From a theoretical perspective, why might this be so?
3. What are the three major areas of treatment for substance addiction, according to Sims? Discuss some of the approaches to treatment from each of these perspectives.
4. What does Sims mean by the statement, "In institutional- or community-based corrections, the realization that recovery from substance abuse is a step-up/step-down/step-up process is critical"?

REFERENCES

Babor, T.F., Kranzler, H.R., & Lauerman, R.J. (1989). Early detection of harmful alcohol consumption: Comparison of clinical, laboratory, and self-report screening procedures. *Addictive Behaviors, 14,* 139-157.

Bandura, A. (1977). *Social learning theory.* Englewood Cliffs, NJ: Prentice Hall.

Blum K., Sheridan, P.J., Wood, R.C., Braverman, E.R., Chen, T.J., & Cummings, D.E. (1995). Dopamine D_2 receptor gene variants: Association and linkage studies in impulsive-addictive-compulsive behavior. *Pharmacogenetics, 5,* 121-141.

Brewer, C. (1993). Recent developments in disulfiram treatment. *Alcohol and Alcoholism, 28,* 383-395.

Brook, J.S., Brook, D.W., Gordon, A.S., Whiteman, M., & Cohen, P. (1990). The psychosocial etiology of adolescent drug use: A family interactional approach. *Genetic, Social, and General Psychology Monographs, 116,* 111-267.

Cooney, N.L., Kadden, R.M., Litt, M.D., & Getter, H. (1991). Matching alcoholics to coping skills or interactional therapies: Two-year follow-up results. *Journal of Consulting and Clinical Psychology, 59,* 598-601.

Ellis, A., McInerney, J.F., DiGuiseppe, R., & Yeager, R.J. (1988). *Rational-emotive therapy with alcoholics and substance abusers.* New York: Pergamon.

Federal Bureau of Prisons. (1999, January). *Substance abuse and treatment programs in the Federal Bureau of Prisons: Report to Congress.* Washington, DC: U.S. Department of Justice.

Greenson, R.R. (1967). *The technique and practice of psychoanalysis.* New York: International Universities Press.

Hawkins, J.D. & Weis, J.G. (1985). The social development model: An integrated approach to delinquency prevention. *Journal of Primary Prevention, 6,* 73-97.

Hull, C. (1943). *Principles of behavior.* New York: Appleton-Century-Crofts.

Hull, J. (1987). Self-awareness model. In H.T. Blane & K.E. Leonard (Eds.), *Psychological theories of drinking and alcoholism* (pp. 272-304). New York: Guilford.

Jung, J. (2001). *Psychology of alcohol and other drugs: A research perspective.* Thousand Oaks, CA: Sage.

MacAndrew, C. & Edgerton, R.B. (1969). *Drunken comportment: A social explanation.* Chicago: Aldine.

Miller, W.R. (1995). Increasing motivation for change. In R.K. Hester & W.R. Miller (Eds.), *Handbook of alcoholism treatment approaches: Effective alternatives* (2nd ed.) (pp. 89-104). Needham Heights, MA: Allyn and Bacon.

National Drug Court Institute. (2002, April). *Methadone maintenance and other pharmacotherapeutic interventions in the treatment of opiod dependence* (Vol. 3, No. 1). Alexandria, VA: National Drug Court Institute.

Office of National Drug Control Policy. (2001). *Drug treatment in the criminal justice system.* Washington, DC: U.S. Government Printing Office.

Pomerleau, O., Pertschuk, M., Adkins, D., & Brady, J.P. (1978). A comparison of behavioral and traditional treatment for middle income problem drinkers. *Journal of Behavioral Medicine, 1,* 187-200.

Prochaska, J., DiClemente, C., & Norcross, J. (1992). In search of how people change: Applications to addictive behaviors. *American Psychologist, 47,* 1102-1114.

Rawson, R., Obert, J., McCann, M., & Varinelli-Casey, P. (1993). Relapse prevention models for substance abuse treatment. *Psychotherapy, 30,* 284-298.

Ryan, R.M., Plant, R.W., & O'Malley, S. (1995). Initial motivations for alcohol treatment: Relations with patient characteristics, treatment involvement, and dropout. *Addictive Behaviors, 20,* 279-297.

Selzer, M.L. (1971). The Michigan Alcohol Screening Test: The quest for a new diagnostic instrument. *American Journal of Psychiatry, 27,* 1653-1658.

Sher, K.J. (1991). *Children of alcoholics: A critical approach of theory and research.* Chicago: Chicago University Press.

Storgaard, H., Nielsen, S.D., & Gluud, C. (1994). The validity of the Michigan Alcoholism Screening Test (MAST). *Alcohol and Alcoholism, 29,* 493-502.

Tarter, R.E., Alterman, A.I., & Edwards, K.L. (1985). Vulnerability to alcoholism in men: A behavior-genetic perspective. *Journal of Studies on Alcohol, 46,* 329-356.

Tarter, R.E., Moss, H., Arria, A.M., Mezzich, A.C., & Vanyukov, M.M. (1992). The psychiatric diagnosis of alcoholism: Critique and proposed reformulation. *Alcoholism, Clinical and Experimental Research, 16,* 106-121.

Taxman, F.S., Silverman, R.S., & Bouffard, J.A. (2000). *Residential substance abuse treatment (RSAT) in prison: Evaluation of the Maryland RSAT program.* College Park, MD: University of Maryland.

Volpicelli, J.R., Clay, K.L., Watson, N.T., & Volpicelli, L.A. (1995). Naltrexone and the treatment of alcohol dependence. *Alcohol Health & Research World, 18*(4), 272-278.

Chapter 2

Predictors of Success and Failure in Correctional-Based Treatment Programs

James W. Golden
Barbara Sims

Just as is the case with any type of rehabilitation or treatment program in the correctional setting, evaluating either institutional- or community-based substance abuse treatment programs can be problematic. Quite often, programs are not implemented the way they were intended to function or they quite simply fail to reach a significant number of the substance-abusing client population. As Farabee et al. (1999) point out, problems with successful implementation leave treatment programs open to incorrect assumptions about their ability to reduce relapses and recidivism; they suggest that program administrators work with key stakeholders (treatment providers, correctional staff, and policymakers) to reduce the negative consequences of improper implementation and other barriers to effective programming.

In spite of the problems with program implementation, the corrections literature has begun to report the successes and failures of substance abuse treatment programs. At a 1997 conference devoted to the study of treating substance abuse in the *community* correctional setting, for example, the International Community Corrections Association heard from several experts in the field, all pointing toward various models that held some promise for success (Latessa, 1999). These models included the use of adequate and appropriate assessment tools, the use of an integrated approach that calls for the simultaneous treatment of co-occurring disorders (both substance abuse and mental health issues), and the use of a cognitive-behavioral model to prevent relapse in the community environment (Latessa, 1999).

In the institutional setting, Simpson, Wexler, and Inciardi (1999), in a meta-analysis of published evaluations of substance abuse treatment programs in the correctional setting, discovered the effectiveness of several programs, including the residential therapeutic community (TC) program, and the ineffectiveness of others, such as boot camps or group counseling. Also showing promise in the attempt to assist offenders overcome the abuse of substances were methadone maintenance treatment programs, twelve-step programs, substance abuse education programs, and cognitive-behavioral therapy models (Simpson et al., 1999).

In the corrections literature is a subsection of studies that alert treatment providers as well as correctional managers to a variety of risks associated with failure in substance abuse treatment programs. The purpose of this chapter is to describe these risks and the importance of addressing them. These risks include the following:

1. a past history of mental health problems;
2. low education levels and accompanying negative self-concepts;
3. gender-specific risks;
4. the dynamics of the group setting;
5. inadequate time in treatment; and
6. an absence of adequate and appropriate postrelease aftercare.

HISTORY OF MENTAL HEALTH PROBLEMS

Offenders with a history of mental health problems who are not properly evaluated prior to placement in treatment are much more likely to drop out of programs due to increased levels of depression and higher levels of anxiety (Moos, Finney, & Moos, 2000; Hiller, Knight, & Simpson, 1999b). Jung (2001) reports a finding of antisocial personality disorders in 15 to 50 percent of alcoholics, for example. This disorder, especially true for males, includes sensation-seeking behaviors coupled with underachievement and a history of childhood misconduct (Jung, 2001). If these past behaviors are not addressed in the treatment setting, along with programs intended to lead the individual to a recognition of his or her problems with substance abuse, treatment of the latter is not likely to be successful. Turning to alcohol and/or other drugs is quite often a means of escaping the deep, dark hole of depression. Specific measures should be taken to ensure that offenders with such histories are placed in proper group settings, especially in light of findings that attention to this particular aspect of treatment can be effective at increasing the success of substance abuse treatment programs (Walters, Heffron, Whitaker, & Dial, 1992).

LOW EDUCATION LEVELS AND NEGATIVE SELF-CONCEPT

Offenders with lower educational levels also appear to be at risk for failing in a substance abuse treatment program, often as a result of poor self-image (Weinberg, 2000) or because of lower retention level (Grella, Vandana, & Hser, 2000). Specialized approaches unique to the needs of these offenders have proven to be quite successful in comparison with traditional approaches. Motivational programs, for example, that instill a sense of confidence in offenders have been found to positively impact individuals' successful completion of treatment (Blankenship, Dansereau, & Simpson, 1999).

Concept mapping has also shown to improve the success rate of substance abuse treatment programs. In this type of activity, specific concepts are outlined and graphically represented so that each concept can be addressed by the group. Retention of information is improved due to the concrete representation of the abstract concepts covered in the program (Pitre, Dees, Dansereau, & Simpson, 1997). In a study by Pitre et al. (1997), offenders who participated in this type of program reported that they worked harder in treatment with their counselors and other group members because of their feelings of inclusion in the process. They also reported an increase in meaningful discussion due to an increased focus on the program curriculum (Pitre et al., 1997).

Hands-on activities and games that are used to represent and teach concepts in substance abuse treatment programs have also proven to be of greater success for offenders with low educational levels. Blankenship et al. (1999) found that group activities in these formats, and with inmates with low education levels, seem to be more conducive to success than one-on-one sessions with individual counselors.

GENDER-SPECIFIC RISKS

Females have been found to be at a higher risk of failure in substance abuse treatment programs than are their male counterparts (Rhodes et al., 2000). In a study performed by the Federal Bureau of Prisons, 75 percent of male inmates graduated from the substance abuse treatment program, while only 58 percent of the females met with success (Pelissier et al., 1998). Whereas 5 percent of male inmates dropped out of the program voluntarily, 8 percent of female inmates did so; and 7 percent of male inmates, compared to 10 percent of female inmates, were ejected from substance abuse treatment programs due to disciplinary infractions (Pelissier et al., 1998).

These findings suggest that more needs to be done when it comes to developing and implementing programs that are specific to females. As Shearer, Myers, and Ogan (2001) point out, the correctional field has begun to develop adequate theories and treatment models for addressing the gender-specific needs of the female correctional client, but much more needs to be done. It is apparent, they argue, that the needs of females differ greatly from those of male clients. Within the female inmate population, for example, Shearer et al. (2001) discovered significant differences related to resistance to treatment based on ethnic and cultural differences, with black and Hispanic females more resistant than white females. They conclude that the hiring and training of counselors who are sensitive to these differences is critical and that better communication in the counselor-client relationship could play a major role in reducing the number of treatment dropouts or failures in this particular population.

Overall, however, and when it comes to treating the substance-addicted female, Shearer et al. (2001) suggest that correctional managers find assistance in the human relations school of administration, getting back to the basics of the construction of an open environment in which counselors engage in reflective listening. Attention should be paid to verbal and nonverbal cues alike, reassuring the female client that she can depend on being heard without being judged for her comments or past behaviors. Although not a panacea for the cessation of substance abuse among the female correctional client, reducing resistance to treatment does appear to be an important first step in that direction.

DYNAMICS OF THE GROUP SETTING

What has been shown almost universally is that when group dynamic problems are solved prior to institution of a treatment regimen, offenders report a higher level of self-efficacy and a reduced propensity toward criminal behavior following release (Hiller et al., 1999b). According to Moos et al. (2000), placing offenders in the group setting whose characteristics differ can cause interpersonal problems that can be extremely detrimental to the success of a substance abuse treatment program. Because of these differences, Moos et al. (2000) strongly encourage clinicians to consider them when referring correctional clients to treatment groups.

Some problems of group dynamics, such as offender education level, cannot be solved, so alternative measures such as specialized group placement must be utilized. Hiller et al. (1999b) have found a link between treatment program failure and cognitive problems, including concentration and memory levels. Individuals who suffer from an inability to think clearly about their substance-abusing behaviors quite often develop a type of interpersonal distress when placed in a group setting that is not conducive to this particular personality disorder (Hiller et al., 1999b).

Similarly, social conformity, or the ability to interact with others absent conflict, should also be recognized and dealt with prior to placement in the group setting. Hiller et al. (1999b) have found that deviant peer groups with antisocial characteristics contribute to failure of substance abuse treatment programs. These types of group dynamics make it difficult for treatment coordinators to establish a favorable rapport with their clients, and prohibit positive and gainful progress for even those offenders who want to be in the programs and who hope to derive success from their time spent in treatment (Hiller et al., 1999b).

LENGTH OF TIME IN TREATMENT

As Jung (2001) cautions, attempts to measure the impact of length of time in any substance abuse treatment program should be undertaken with much care. All too often, evaluations of this nature are conducted absent a control group, or groups, with no comparisons made between and/or among groups at varied posttreatment time spans. Welte, Hynes, Sokolov, and Lyons (1981) have, however, found greater success among groups who underwent treatment in programs of a greater duration than programs of a shorter time frame. In the correctional institution setting, measures in a study by McCusker et al. (1997) at eighteen months after completion of a substance abuse treatment program indicated that those in three-month programs were subjected to more intense treatment regimens than those in the six-month programs. The hurried pace of the shorter programs, however, did not allow satisfactory retention of the concepts presented, as the longer, six-month programs allowed. The authors concluded that those offenders in the three-month programs could benefit from an additional six months; however, those in the six-month programs would not likely see any benefits from extended treatment experiences (McCusker et al., 1997).

One six-month full-service residential community program in Florida, referred to as a nonsecure drug treatment (NSDT) program, appears to be successful in preventing relapse. Bryant (2000) reports that these types of programs are found throughout the state and are designed for severely addicted correctional clients. Kept in the community, these individuals undergo treatment in programs that have been contracted out by the department of corrections to private providers. NSDT programs are unique in that they are longer in duration than most treatment programs, with attendees reporting that an almost lifetime habit of substance abuse is not readily turned around in the typical twenty-eight-day programs (Bryant, 2000). The six-month program consists of intensive drug and/or alcohol treatment coupled with equally intensive efforts at assisting the individual to find and maintain employment. The treatment component primarily is grounded in addiction education, life-management skills, and relapse prevention, with all three of these components teaching the individual to recognize certain triggers for addictive behavior and how to avoid them. Bryant (2000) reports statistics indicating that 63 percent of the more than 10,000 offenders who have participated in Florida's NSDT programs never return to prison or correctional supervision.

It is not reaching to argue that the greater the duration of treatment, combined with supervision by the corrections community, the greater the likelihood for remaining relapse free. This is particularly true when treatment follows offenders into their local communities once they are released from a secure institution or, if released from a nonsecure community treatment facility, when clients are given some assistance with aftercare needs.

POSTRELEASE AFTERCARE PROGRAMMING

One of the more profound problems with substance abuse treatment program graduates is the readjustment to normal life following release. Additional support would be beneficial as the transition is made. Cost is an issue with transitional residential programs. Private facilities charge an average of $49 per day for a period of approximately 140 days, while short-term stays of up to three months can cost as much as $130 per day (Uziel-Miller, Lyons, Rowland, Conrad, & Kendo, 1999). Government-financed transitional programs may be able to offer similar programs at a reduced cost. In many instances, the benefits far outweigh the costs, such as in the case of individuals with psychological or social problems (Guydish et al., 1999).

Studies have demonstrated that there is a lower risk for rearrest following release for inmates who participated in treatment programs while incarcerated, but this is especially true of offenders who follow their release with a residential, community-based program (Hiller, Knight, & Simpson, 1999a). A study by Hiller et al. (1999a) found that parolees had time to find employment and better residential arrangements if they were involved in a transitional program, receiving support and counseling during this time. They found that those who did receive this type of aftercare programming were significantly less likely to be arrested than those who did not take part in a transitional program (Hiller et al., 1999a).

In the Hiller et al. (1999a) study, those offenders who dropped out of transitional treatment reported that they did so because the institutional- and community-based treatment programs did not complement each other. Treatment programs during incarceration were based on peer group dynamics, while follow-up treatment programs after release were structured to follow a medical model (Hiller et al., 1999a). This suggests that the same attention to individual needs when it comes to treatment on the inside needs to be given to community correctional clients as they make the transition to life on the outside. To ignore the specific needs of individuals would, in essence, mean a return to the "one size can fit all" model of treatment, an approach that we now know will not work with substance-addicted individuals.

Residential aftercare is also needed to integrate the offender back into society. Living arrangements prior to incarceration serve as an indicator of potential success in a substance abuse treatment program. Those offenders who were homeless before their arrest and subsequent incarceration were more likely to fail completion of a substance abuse treatment program (Moos et al., 2000). Furthermore, offenders who have a history of unemployment have been found to fail completion of substance abuse treatment programs more often than those who had a previously consistent employment history. In a similar vein, assistance in becoming familiar with structure and ordered tasks has been found helpful for the postrelease correctional client (Hiller et al., 1999b). This holistic approach to follow-up support and treatment appears to be critical in the avoidance of relapses into drug and/or alcohol use and the establishment of a more positive daily routine and subsequently a productive, crime-free lifestyle.

SUMMARY AND CONCLUSIONS

The information reported here suggests several possibilities. Substance abuse treatment programs in the correctional setting quite often offer positive benefits to participants, and those offenders that complete programs have a significantly higher likelihood of returning to society as productive and law-abiding individuals. There are drawbacks, however, to each treatment approach, and these problems contribute to the relapse to drug use and criminal activity for certain individuals. Inmates with low educational levels and negative self-concepts are likely to have problems completing a substance abuse treatment program. Those with a history of mental health problems often fail in treatment if special attention is not given to these problems.

Length of time in treatment is another consideration for corrections managers. Programs of a longer duration work better at reducing relapse, but some evidence surfacing suggests that a more intense, accelerated program might be able to accomplish a similar goal. Regardless of type or duration of program however, emphasis must also be placed on postrelease aftercare. Much of the literature reported previously suggests that programming should be placed within the larger context of continuing to meet the specific and individual needs of correctional clients while, at the same time, addressing the more immediate needs of housing and meaningful employment.

Although correctional managers who are faced with budgetary restraints will find it difficult to cater to each inmate's specific needs, we suggest that some measures can be taken to integrate various treatment approaches designed to address a wider variety of presenting problems. The group setting, for example, a widely used treatment approach in correctional settings, could be enhanced by the careful matching of inmates with similar problems and by the simultaneous treatment of identified co-occurring conditions. With the reemergence of the rehabilitative ideal in the 1990s, following on the heels of both a control and incapacitation model of corrections, there was a recognition that a "one size fits all" model of treatment will not work. This is especially true of the substance-addicted offender. Vigdal and Stadler (1996) point out that these individuals are not a homogeneous group, and because they are not, any attempt at rehabilitation will fail if the needs of certain subgroups of the larger population are not met. Mixed modalities of treatment does, of course, call for specialized and experienced staff, and this can be an expensive undertaking. Too, both the treatment industry and correctional managers must be prepared to accept and treat an increasing number of clients, adding additional costs to correctional budgets that are already, in some cases, suffering from growing pains as corrections populations continue to expand (Vigdal & Stadler, 1996).

As previously noted (see the Introduction to this book), it is difficult to draw a straight line between substance abuse and criminal behavior. In the middle of the controversy over this issue, however, some suggest that addiction "serves as a multiplier of crime" (Murray, 1996:90). Although, as argued by Murray (1996), addiction often occurs prior to criminal behavior, it also can serve to increase individuals' involvement in such activity. In the light of the extant research on substance abuse treatment programs in the correctional environment which shows that treatment can work both to reduce relapses into drug and/or alcohol abuse and to reduce criminal offending among this population, it would seem well worth the investment of resources into these programs. The field of corrections appears to have awakened to this fact and is moving in the right direction. The subsequent chapters here address some of the problems and successes encountered with a variety of substance abuse treatment programs within both the institutional and community corrections settings.

DISCUSSION QUESTIONS

1. Why, as Jung (2001) argues, might we find a significant number of individuals diagnosed with antisocial personality disorder among alcoholics?
2. In addition to mental health issues, what other issues need to be taken into account when it comes to developing a treatment program for the substance-addicted individual?
3. Discuss some of the problems that correctional managers are likely to encounter when they attempt to develop and implement substance abuse treatment from a multimodality approach.

REFERENCES

Blankenship, J., Dansereau, D.F., & Simpson, D.D. (1999). Cognitive enhancements of readiness for corrections-based treatment for drug abuse. *The Prison Journal, 79,* 431-455.

Bryant, P.T. (2000). Florida's award-winning nonsecure drug treatment program. *Corrections Today, 62*(3), 98-101.

Farabee, D., Prendergast, M., Cartier, J., Wexler, H., Knight, K., & Anglin, M.D. (1999). Barriers to implementing effective correctional drug treatment programs. *The Prison Journal, 79*(2), 150-162.

Grella, C.E., Vandana, J., & Hser, Y. (2000). Program variation in treatment outcomes among women in residential drug treatment. *Evaluation Review, 24,* 364-383.

Guydish, J., Sorenson, J.L., Chan, M., Bostrom, A., Werdegar, D., & Acampora, A. (1999). A randomized trial comparing day and residential drug abuse treatment: 18-month outcomes. *Journal of Counseling and Clinical Psychology, 67,* 428-434.

Hiller, M.L., Knight, K., & Simpson, D.D. (1999a). Prison-based substance abuse treatment, residential aftercare, and recidivism. *Addiction, 94,* 833-842.

Hiller, M.L., Knight, K., & Simpson, D.D. (1999b). Risk factors that predict dropout from corrections-based treatment for drug abuse. *The Prison Journal, 79,* 411-430.

Jung, J. (2001). *Psychology of alcohol and other drugs: A research perspective.* Thousand Oaks, CA: Sage.

Latessa, E.J. (1999). *Strategic solutions: The International Community Corrections Association examines substance abuse.* Papers delivered at the "What Works" Research Conference, Cleveland, OH, 1997. Arlington, VA: American Corrections Association.

McCusker, J., Bigelow, C., Vickers-Lahti, M., Spotts, D., Garfield, F., & Frost, F. (1997). Planned duration of residential drug abuse treatment: Efficacy versus effectiveness. *Addiction, 92,* 1467-1478.

Moos, R.H., Finney, J.W., & Moos, B.S. (2000). Inpatient substance abuse care and the outcome of subsequent community residential and outpatient care. *Addiction, 95,* 833-846.

Murray, D.W., Jr. (1996). Drug abuse treatment in the Federal Bureau of Prisons: A historical review and assessment of contemporary initiatives. In K.E. Early (Ed.), *Drug treatment behind bars: Prison-based strategies for change* (pp. 88-100). Westport, CT: Praeger.

Pelissier, B., Wallace, S., O'Neil, J.A., Gaes, G.G., Camp, S., Rhodes, W., & Saylor, W. (1998). Federal prison residential drug treatment reduces substance use and arrests after release. Unpublished manuscript. Washington, DC: Federal Bureau of Prisons.

Pitre, U., Dees, S.M., Dansereau, D.F., & Simpson, D.D. (1997). Mapping techniques to improve substance abuse treatment in criminal justice settings. *Journal of Drug Issues, 27,* 431-444.

Rhodes, W., Pelissier, B., Gaes, G., Saylor, W., Camp, S., & Wallace, S. (2000). Alternative solutions to the problem of selection bias in analysis of federal residential drug treatment programs. Unpublished manuscript. Washington, DC: Federal Bureau of Prisons.

Shearer, R.A., Myers, L.B., & Ogan, G.D. (2001). Treatment resistance and ethnicity among female offenders in substance abuse treatment programs. *The Prison Journal, 81*(1), 55-72.

Simpson, D.D., Wexler, H.K., & Inciardi, J.C. (1999). Drug treatment outcomes for correctional settings. *The Prison Journal, 79*(4), 379-445.

Uziel-Miller, N.D., Lyons, J.S., Rowland, B., Conrad, K.J., & Kendo, J. (1999). A safe haven: An innovative approach to residential treatment of substance abuse. *American Journal of Public Health, 89,* 1430-1431.

Vigdal, G.L. & Stadler, D.W. (1996). Assessment, client treatment matching, and managing the substance abusing offender. In K.E. Early (Ed.), *Drug treatment behind bars: Prison-based strategies for change* (pp. 17-43). Westport, CT: Praeger.

Walters, G.D., Heffron, M., Whitaker, D., & Dial, S. (1992). The CHOICE Program: A comprehensive residential treatment program for drug-involved federal offenders. *International Journal of Offender Therapy and Comparative Criminology, 36,* 21-29.

Weinberg, D. (2000). "Out there": The ecology of addiction in drug abuse treatment discourse. *Social Problems, 47*(4), 606-622.

Welte, J., Hynes, G., Sokolov, J., & Lyons, J.P. (1981). Effect of length of stay in inpatient alcoholism treatment on outcome. *Journal of Studies on Alcohol, 42,* 483-491.

Chapter 3

Treatment Motivation Characteristics of Offenders Who Abuse Substances

Robert A. Shearer

For more than two decades, programs for offenders who abuse substances have been a traditional part of institutional corrections. The importance and scope of substance abuse treatment programs have varied from time to time and program to program. Historically, only a small percentage of the offender population has been involved in these programs (Austin, 1998).

As substance abuse treatment programs have evolved, a greater interest has been developing in some of the clinical characteristics of offenders, parallel to concerns about program effectiveness. Correctional managers have, understandably, been concerned about program effectiveness, but recently somewhat fragmented and scattered research results are providing some worthwhile clinical directives for increasing program efficiency. It would, therefore, seem beneficial to correctional managers to pull together the results of these research initiatives into some meaningful conclusions for managerial decision making.

This discussion is an attempt to present the available knowledge concerning one of the several clinical characteristics of offenders who abuse substances. Specifically, motivation to participate in substance abuse treatment is the concern here and not offender characteristics such as risk tendencies to recidivate or criminal thinking and behavior. These additional offender characteristics have certainly been an important part of recent research endeavors, and they are important considerations for correctional decision making. The focus of this discussion, however, is to synthesize the information available on motivation to enter treatment programs in corrections and motivation for behavior change once the offender is undergoing treatment for substance abuse. Hopefully, this synthesis will be useful for managers in both institutional and community corrections.

Some important points, related to the previously mentioned fragmented and disconnected research results, should preface the task of providing this synthesis. First, the various approaches to motivation are not presented in an order of importance, even though some have been more extensive than others. Conclusions as to their importance are left to the reader and each manager's particular needs. Second, most of the research is experimental at this time and some studies are based on limited samples, so caution is recommended in drawing anything but tentative conclusions. Third, the various approaches to offender motivation use different terms to explain the characteristic. They may be explaining the same characteristic. On the other hand, they may be explaining different characteristics or common parts of the same characteristic. The sophistication level in the literature does not seem to have reached a point where the terminology or theory is consistent across various approaches to offender motivation. This needs to be understood from the beginning. This and future discussions will contribute toward rectifying this troubling condition as more work is done in the field. Nevertheless, some interesting and creative work has been advancing our understanding of treatment motivation. These advances have focused on treatment motivation both in and out of correctional settings.

COMPLIANCE VERSUS INTERNALIZATION

One of the earliest discussions of client motivation was the distinction between compliance and internalization made by Kelman (1971) and subsequently discussed by Lewis, Dana, and Blevins (1994) in the context of group work. *Compliance* involves conformity to the wishes, demands, or influence of another person or group. The client exhibits the desired behavior not because of a belief in the usefulness of the change but because of external rewards or punishments. Compliant behavior produces superficial and politically correct actions. It means doing and saying the expected to reduce environmental pressure from the group. On the other hand, *internalization* occurs when individuals actually believe that new behaviors will be useful to them. Internalized behavior is intrinsically rewarding to the person.

One of the key concepts of the compliance and internalization discussion is what Kelman (1971) refers to as "surveillance by the influencing agent." He indicates that behavior exhibited under the conditions of compliance is likely to be performed only under conditions in which the individual is being watched by the coercive agent. The important question for correctional treatment is how much of the adopted behavior will be performed when surveillance is eliminated.

Connors, Donovan, and DiClemente (2001) indicate similar characteristics of individuals who are in treatment as a result of compliance. These individuals seek clinical treatment solely to placate others. They are not truly ready to change their abuse of substances. In addition, these individuals can be described as defensive, passive about their drug use, avoiding steps to change their behavior, unaware of a problem, and feeling pressured by other people. The primary characteristic of these individuals is that they are not considering or thinking about changing their behavior. A more thorough discussion of this lack of motivation to change behavior appears in a subsequent section concerning a theoretical model of behavior change.

Treatment compliance has also played a major role in motivation in therapeutic communities. DeLeon (1994) has identified compliance as the first stage in a resident's attitudes toward therapeutic communities. Residents of such communities move from the first stage of compliance, to conformity, to commitment. In the first stage, residents simply adhere to the rules to avoid negative consequences. In the second stage, residents adhere to the norms of the therapeutic community to avoid loss of approval or disaffiliation. Finally, residents develop a sense of commitment to change destructive attitudes and behaviors. If a resident makes it to the final stage without leaving prematurely, he or she is highly likely to be crime free or drug free in the future. Consequently, DeLeon (1994) sees compliance as a result of the legal force to get offenders into treatment until they internalize the value and goals of recovery. Unfortunately, research as to how a person moves through these stages and what actually occurs in therapeutic communities has not been extensively studied. The theory of compliance is one of dragging their bodies into treatment and hoping their hearts and minds will follow. Unfortunately, we do not know how or for what individuals this works.

Compliance is a particularly attractive motivational characteristic of treatment programs for correctional managers. First, compliance fits quite well into the authoritarian model of the courts, probation, and prison. The criminal justice system operates on legal judgments and directives to satisfy the courts. A determination of the individual's willingness to cooperate is not a typical factor in mandated treatment. Consequently, many individuals who are ordered to attend treatment do not have any real intentions to change their behavior (Connors et al., 2001). Second, compliant behavior is considerably easier to document and monitor than internalized behavior. Internalized behavior change is more subjective and may not emerge until a later date, well after program completion and release. It is a major task for correctional managers and clinicians to ensure, for example, program attendance and participation so that the integrity of the treatment program is not compromised. It may be too much to ask correctional managers to make a major effort to determine if the behavior they are observing is real or fake.

The important lesson from research on motivation is that there is a difference between *motivation for treatment* and *motivation for authentic behavior change* (DiClemente, 1999). The former typically involves short-term compliance and the latter a major lifestyle change.

Coerced versus Voluntary Treatment

The previous discussion shows that there are some important questions about the role of coercion in motivation for substance abuse treatment. The central concern is the amount of motivation that is necessary when individuals are coerced to begin treatment rather than voluntarily choosing to stop their substance abuse (Stevens & Smith, 2001). Coerced drug treatment has been praised (Satel, 2000) and cursed (Shearer, 2000). This paradox leaves correctional managers in a dilemma as to the role of coercion in substance abuse treatment.

This dilemma has been developing for a number of years because it has become common practice in the United States for offenders to be ordered to undergo counseling. This practice is variously referred to as "coerced treatment," "court-ordered treatment," "mandated treatment," "involuntary treatment," or "compulsory treatment." In any case, the practice constitutes some degree of involuntary counseling and a guaranteed caseload for a counselor. In addition, the practice may also include one or more of the following conditions:

1. Clients may not think they have a need for counseling.
2. Clients may not actually have a problem.
3. Clients do not choose their therapist.
4. Clients cannot change their therapist.
5. Clients cannot freely terminate counseling.
6. Because of the serious consequences for leaving counseling, clients may be forced to consider compliance to avoid these consequences.
7. Clients may be agreeing to enter a counseling relationship or treatment program without sufficient information about the relationship or program.

The degree to which these elements exist in the practice of coerced counseling determines the extent to which treatment is "coerced" or "compulsory." Not all offenders who are ordered to go to counseling, of course, are reluctant to enter counseling and may welcome the opportunity to enter into a relationship or to participate in a program that will help improve their lives or personal problems. Furthermore, many offenders participate in other forms of treatment in addition to counseling. Substantial psychiatric literature and a large body of case law covers the right to refuse treatment, even when treatment has been court ordered (Winick, 1997). Consequently, coerced substance abuse counseling is the focus of the debate, and not the delivery of psychiatric and mental health services that tend to be viewed under a broader canopy of correctional treatment.

The issue of coerced counseling reached a peak in the late 1980s and was focused primarily on drug abusers who were required to attend treatment programs. The discussions of coerced treatment seem to have been stimulated by several research reports appearing at that time concerning the effectiveness of coerced treatment. During the time the discussion was at its height, several writers questioned coerced treatment on philosophical, clinical, and legal grounds (Platt, Buhringer, Kaplan, & Brown, 1988; Rosenthal, 1988; Boyd, Millard, & Webster, 1985). On the other hand, two U.S. government publications clearly explain the other side of the issue. "Excluding people from treatment merely because of a lack of readiness, based on denial, would mean that the treatment process would never begin for many" (Inciardi, 1994:18), and "Few chronic addicts will enter treatment without some type of external motivation and that legal coercion is as justified as any other treatment motivation" (Vigdal, 1995:9). Inciardi (1994:18) further notes:

> Among clients mandated to treatment from the criminal justice system, it is unusual for a client to be genuinely enthusiastic about entering treatment. Most clients are not ready, do not want to be in treatment, and do not like it.

Typically though, correctional clients perceive treatment as a more attractive alternative than incarceration. The dilemma presented by coerced treatment is that others see the need for treatment for an individual, but the individual does not see the need. In traditional counseling practice, clients are ready when they "own" the problem and accept the need for treatment. Consequently, the unique strategy of coerced treatment is to create extrinsic pressure on the person, through legal means, in order to create a fear of incarceration.

Currently, this strategy is in operation at the local, state, and national level where offenders are court ordered to enter residential treatment facilities, in-prison therapeutic communities, and community outpatient counseling programs for substance abuse problems. The earlier cautions were either unknown or unheeded as the field of substance abuse treatment has become a criminal justice problem so that coerced counseling has become quite commonplace and widely practiced.

Satel (2000) has looked at the practice of coercion in a wide variety of settings, including therapeutic communities, prison programs, drug courts, and prison diversion programs. She found strong evidence for the effectiveness of coerced treatment programs. Her conclusion was that "addicts need not be internally motivated at the onset of treatment in order to benefit from it" (Satel, 2000:1). Consequently, there is a strong case for the use of coercion in treatment settings.

Part of the problem of coerced treatment lies in the meaning of the word *treatment.* If treatment means drug testing and monitoring along with court surveillance, then few problems arise in the case of coerced treatment. If coerced treatment includes counseling or psychotherapy, then the practice is very troublesome on several grounds. First, none of the major theories of counseling or psychotherapy are designed or developed for involuntary clients. They assume voluntary participation. Virtually all professionally trained counselors know this, so the professional integrity of the counselor in a coerced relationship would certainly be in question. If the counselor is an amateur or untrained volunteer, then the question has little relevance because we would not expect positive outcomes beyond chance successes if we truly support the value of trained professional counselors. Second, the reported successes of coerced treatment programs have little value other than alleviating political pressure for treatment success and cost-effectiveness, because few process evaluations have been conducted on coerced treatment programs. In other words, we know something is working in some programs to reduce recidivism; we simply do not know what it is. Without program replication, we cannot make progress in the field.

Finally, the most serious challenge to the practice of coerced treatment is the clearly stated codes of ethics of virtually all of the psychology, counseling, and social work professional organizations. The foundation of ethical practice is freedom of choice and informed consent. Coerced psychological intervention in an individual's life suggests the practice of brainwashing because it consists of pressure to change thoughts, values, or attitudes under the threat of serious legal consequences. In addition to ethical considerations about how coerced counseling affects the offender, a perhaps greater concern is how it affects the counselor who is practicing a profession in an arena where there are serious theoretical, empirical, and ethical threats to professionalism (Shearer, 2000).

Intrinsic versus Extrinsic Motivation

Another approach to the question about how motivated an individual is to change substance abuse or to enter treatment focuses on characteristics of the individual. This approach suggests that an important dimension is the locus of motivation (Donovan & Rosengren, 1999). According to this approach, what should be looked at are the reasons an individual is seeking to change behavior or to enter treatment. Is the motivation originating in *intrinsic* factors or *extrinsic* demands and pressures? Are there inner or external reasons for seeking change or treatment?

The research and theory on extrinsic and intrinsic motivation provides some helpful guidelines to correctional managers. First, most individuals seek treatment initially in response to external pressure rather than some form of internal revelation. Second, substance abusers indicate they are motivated to seek treatment for a variety of private and social factors. Private factors include health and self-control concerns. Social factors include fear of getting into trouble with the legal system or losing a job. Third, clients high in both intrinsic and extrinsic motivation are the most successful in treatment. They show the best attendance in treatment and they tend not to drop out of treatment. Fourth, substance abuse clients low in internal motivation are likely to be the poorest candidates for treatment. Fifth, it appears, though research is not conclusive, that the role of substance abuse treatment is to shift client motivation from extrinsic to intrinsic. This shift is consistent with the majority of the major counseling and psychotherapy theories. Finally, measures of motivation should incorporate these different concepts of motivation because research results suggest it is a multivariate construct (Donovan & Rosengren, 1999).

Readiness to Change

One of the most thoroughly researched and widely used approaches to motivation offers correctional managers a new approach to behavior change. The transtheoretical model (TTM) (Prochaska & DiClemente, 1986) and the stages of change model are both based on the notion that individuals are located at different stages and move through the stages in a process of change. The TTM is currently being used by professionals around the world as a model of behavior change and treatment interventions (Velasquez, Maurer, Crouch, & DiClemente, 2001).

Most of the research completed by Prochaska and colleagues (Prochaska & DiClemente, 1986; Prochaska, DiClemente, & Norcross, 1992) on addictions was completed near the end of the twentieth century. To ensure their interventions were sensitive to clients' level of readiness to change, they developed and validated a self-report measure, the University of Rhode Island Change Assessment (URICA), using various samples of individuals with addictive behaviors such as smoking and substance abuse.

Four stages of change were identified: precontemplation, contemplation, action, and maintenance. In the *precontemplation* stage, the individual is not even considering the possibility of change. Individuals in this stage typically perceive that they are being coerced into treatment to satisfy someone else's need. The *contemplation* stage is characterized by ambivalence. This stage indicates that individuals may simultaneously, or in rapid alternation, consider or reject reasons to change. Individuals in the *action* stage have made a commitment to change and are engaging in actions to bring about change. Typically, at this stage they are involved in therapy or other forms of treatment. Finally, individuals in the *maintenance* stage are working to sustain the significant changes they have made and are actively working to prevent relapse (DiClemente & Porches, 1998). This model highlights the importance of treatment readiness and is consistent with the responsivity concept. In addition, the URICA provides a method for assessing treatment readiness and responsivity with offenders for research and treatment planning purposes, but the scale is still being validated for research use.

Correctional treatment programs are frequently designed as action-oriented treatment and self-help programs, but correctional counselors and administrators are disappointed when only a small percentage of addicted people indicate an interest in the program or stay with the program through completion (Prochaska et al., 1992). Resnick and Rozensky (1996) indicate that we cannot treat people with a precontemplation profile as if they were ready for action interventions and expect them to stay in the program. The most effective strategy to promote retention is matching interventions to stage of change.

Silverstein (1997) found that legally coerced substance abuse clients were less likely to participate in treatment to the same extent as voluntary clients. His research tended to support observations by clinicians that coerced clients continue to lag behind those not legally coerced, even though they make incrementally equivalent progress in changing their behavior. Apparently, coerced counseling is more a problem of *efficiency* than *effectiveness* because, as Silverstein (1997) found, court-mandated clients enter treatment at a significantly earlier stage in the change process than do non–court mandated clients.

URICA RESEARCH

Since its development as a measure of treatment readiness in smokers, the URICA has continued to produce studies of motivation to change. Recently, the URICA has been used to study methadone patients (Belding, Iguchi, & Lamb, 1996), sex offenders (Serin & Kennedy, 1997), alcoholics (Willoughby & Edens, 1996), adolescent psychiatric patients (Greenstein, Franklin, & McGuffin, 1999), court-mandated substance abusers (Silverstein, 1997), and smokers (Norman, Velicer, Fava, & Prochaska, 1998).

The psychometric properties of the URICA have been studied to determine "fakeability" (Brigham, 1996), validity (Belding, Iguchi, & Lamb, 1996), predictive utility (Willoughby & Edens, 1997), concurrent validity (Rothfleisch, 1998), and reliability (McConnaughy, Prochaska, & Velieer, 1983; McConnaughy, DiClemente, Prochaska, & Velicer, 1989; DiClemente & Hughes, 1990). In general, the instrument continues to demonstrate strong properties as a measure of change motivation.

The URICA has occasionally been used to identify an individual's location in one of the stages of change by identifying the scale on which an individual scores highest (Prochaska, Norcross, Fowler, & Follick, 1992). On the other hand, the recommended purpose of the URICA is to identify specific stage profiles characteristic of transitions between the four basic stages of change or to identify subtypes of individuals within a stage of change (Velicer, Hughes, Fava, Prochaska, & DiClemente, 1995).

These profiles of change have been developed for a diverse group of problem behaviors, such as smoking, cocaine use, weight control, delinquency, exercising, and condom use (Resnick & Rozensky, 1996). Specifically, McConnaughy et al. (1983) developed nine clusters and then in 1989, in a replication study, developed eight clusters for clients entering psychotherapy. Simourd and O'Connor (2000) used the eight-cluster approach, from the replication study, to classify probationers. They were able to classify 70 percent of the cases in the study in the eight clusters, which was 20 percent lower than the rate in two earlier studies. Finally, DiClemente and Hughes (1990) developed profiles of change in alcoholism treatment by identifying specific clusters within the stages of change. These studies used the statistical procedure of cluster analysis in their research in order to reduce a sample of cases to a few statistically significant groups. These clusters were based on differences and similarities across the stages of the URICA. In other words, they wanted to know if patterns would emerge in the four scales of the URICA that would indicate a profile of motivation, i.e., a cluster that might reappear across various populations of addicted subjects.

The clusters they identified were participation, uninvolved, contemplation, ambivalent, and precontemplation. The *participation* cluster is characterized by low precontemplation scores, high contemplation scores, and high action and maintenance scores. High or low scores are defined as being above or below the mean, respectively. The *uninvolved* cluster is characterized by low precontemplation, contemplation, action, and maintenance scores. The *contemplation* cluster indicates precontemplation scale scores below the mean, with contemplation scale scores above the mean and action scale scores below the mean. The *ambivalent* cluster is characterized by precontemplation, contemplation, action, and maintenance scale scores above the mean. The *precontemplation* cluster shows precontemplation scale scores above the mean and the other three scale scores below the mean.

In a recent study by Shearer and Ogan (2002a), it was found that two-thirds of a sample of substance-abusing offenders were not ready to change as indicated by the high scores on precontemplation. In addition, it was found that the profile of change in the sample indicated a motivation for change characterized by the ambivalent cluster. These offenders were considering reasons to change but were also considering reasons to reject change.

The most important conclusion from Shearer and Ogan's (2002b) study was that about one-third of the offenders were ready to change their behavior. It is, perhaps, these offenders who should be the focus of more active treatment interventions and valuable correctional resources.

RESISTANCE TO TREATMENT

The final approach to treatment motivation has been studied by individuals who are curious about the phenomenon of resistance to counseling or treatment. Their research looks at barriers to motivation. As discussed earlier, counseling in the correctional setting rarely involves voluntary clients, so resistance to counseling by offenders is common (Romig & Gruenke, 1991; Harris, 2001; Walters, 2001). Miller (1985) indicates that motivation is the flip side of denial and resistance (cited in Connors et al., 2001). This description of the phenomenon may be misleading because it suggests a dichotomous relationship, but the relationship may, in fact, be ordinal. In other words, there may be degrees of motivation and resistance, ranging from highly motivated to extremely resistant, with various levels in between.

Resistance to counseling is a clinical phenomenon that has been described by a multitude of definitions which differ along certain dimensions. Some of these descriptions have been identified as precontemplation (Prochaska et al., 1992), reluctance (Cullari, 1996), denial (Rothschild, 1995), psychoanalytic resistance (Cullari, 1996), general resistance (Rothschild, 1995), substance abuse questionnaire (SAQ)-resistance (Behavior Data Systems, 1985), responsivity (Serin & Kennedy, 1997), and amenability (Palmer, 1994).

As can be seen in the previous discussion, the motivational picture is complicated by both specific and general definitions of resistance in the literature. General or specific, active or passive, the importance of resistance as a motivational factor is very critical in substance abuse counseling and treatment programs. Because resistance is an important motivational factor, the correctional treatment resistance scale (CTRS) was developed as a method to quantify resistance to substance abuse counseling (Shearer, 1999, in press). The CTRS has demonstrated initial promise as a psychometric instrument that can be used in screening offenders for participation in substance abuse counseling programs. First, the CTRS has shown respectable reliability across the entire instrument and among the various subscales. Second, the validity of the CTRS is supported by factor analysis which tends to indicate that the instrument consists of three components. The first two components are not as easy to identify as the third component, but they do have some conceptually consistent items.

Component 1 seems to be measuring resistance to treatment originating in cynicism about prison counseling and denial of any need for counseling. The highest loading in this component was the item which indicated that the subject thought that prison counseling was "useless bull sessions." This item accounted for over half of the variance. On the other hand, several other items loaded on this component, so the item does not completely consist of these concepts.

Component 2 seems to be measuring distrust of counselors and a reluctance to discuss personal problems. The highest loading was on the item that concerned sharing personal problems with a counselor. Isolation and low self-disclosure also seem to be a part of this component.

Component 3 presents a much clearer picture of the concept it is measuring. Three of the five items appeared that were originally on the cultural issues scale. The other two items could be interpreted as cultural issues which would support their loadings on this component. This finding supports the literature of treatment with diverse populations of offenders concerning the importance of cultural issues in treatment readiness.

Using the CTRS, Shearer, Myers, and Ogan (2001) found, in a study of female offenders in substance abuse treatment programs, that resistance was consistent across a variety of treatment groups. They also indicated that elevated resistance scores were observed for black and Hispanic female offenders. The study underscored the importance of cultural and gender diversity in treatment planning and interventions.

Finally, Shearer and Ogan (2002b) studied treatment resistance between voluntary and forced participation for three treatment groups of male offenders. They found that offenders who perceived they had volunteered for treatment were 20 percent less resistant than those who indicated they were forced to participate. Consequently, the perception of voluntary participation may be as important as actual voluntary participation when the latter is an unrealistic arrangement. This is a particularly interesting finding in light of the fact that none of the subjects in the study were in treatment programs on a voluntary basis.

SUMMARY AND CONCLUSIONS

Motivation is a very important element of treatment for offenders who abuse substances. It is an element that appears to play a vital role in the process of breaking an addiction. Questions about the role of motivation by correctional managers are likely to be similar to the questions asked by behavioral scientists and addiction professionals. First, what motivates or prevents offenders from considering quitting their substance abuse? Second, what motivates them to actually try to quit? Third, why is it so difficult to maintain their level of motivation? Finally, how do they stay drug free over a long period of time (Jung, 2001)?

Fortunately, several significant advances have been made in answering some of these questions. Research on motivation and theoretical models of change have been the primary themes of investigation into the answers for these questions. The advances are at varying points of development, but several useful conclusions for correctional managers can be made. It is always risky to synthesize complex technical information, but the goal here is to offer some practical guidelines for correctional managers, without running the risk of oversimplification.

First, short-term compliance is different from genuine behavior change, and correctional managers may have to settle for the more superficial of the two goals. Second, coerced treatment seems to be effective, but not efficient, in reducing recidivism. In addition, it is accompanied by serious research and professional challenges. Third, most offenders are externally pressured into treatment, but a combination of external and internal motivation is preferable for treatment success. Fourth, we know a great deal about how the process of change occurs. Fifth, many offenders are ready to change their behavior. Sixth, we have some excellent instruments, in various stages of development, for measuring treatment motivation or resistance. Finally, motivation for treatment may be culturally driven so that motivation is not only a multidimensional but also a multicultural phenomenon. If motivation is viewed from these perspectives, then treatment planning and interventions are likely to be more successful in reducing relapse and recidivism in the short term and public safety for the long term.

DISCUSSION QUESTIONS

1. Discuss how Shearer, drawing from the previous literature, differentiates between *compliance* and *internalization* when it comes to clients' motivation to enter a substance abuse treatment program.
2. Why does Shearer argue that compliance is an "attractive" motivation characteristic within the correctional environment?

3. Describe the ongoing debate about the benefits, or lack thereof, of coerced treatment. What recommendations does Shearer give to correctional managers when it comes to this critical component of substance abuse treatment?

REFERENCES

Austin, J. (1998). The limits of drug treatment. *Corrections Management Quarterly, 2*(4), 66-74.

Behavior Data Systems, Ltd. (1985). *Substance abuse questionnaire research summary.* Phoenix, AZ: Author.

Belding, M.A., Iguchi, M.Y., & Lamb, R.J. (1996). Stages of change in methadone maintenance: Assessing the convergent validity of two measures. *Psychology of Addictive Behaviors, 10*(3), 157-166.

Boyd, N., Millard, C., & Webster, C.D. (1985). Heroin "treatment" in British Columbia, 1976-1984: Thesis, anthesis, and synthesis. *Canadian Journal of Criminology, 27*(2), 195-208.

Brigham, G.S. (1996). Fakeability of the University of Rhode Island Change Assessment with a substance abuse population. *Dissertation Abstracts International, 57,* 5-13. University Microfilm No. 1419-4217.

Connors, G.J., Donovan, D.M., & DiClemente, C.C. (2001). *Substance abuse treatment and the stages of change.* New York: Guilford.

Cullari, S. (1996). *Treatment resistance: A guide for practitioners.* Boston: Allyn & Bacon.

DeLeon, G. (1994). The therapeutic community: Toward a general theory and model. In F.M. Tims, G. DeLeon, & N. Jainchill (Eds.), *Therapeutic community: Advances in research and application* (pp. 16-53). Rockville, MD: National Institute on Drug Abuse.

DiClemente, C.C. (1999). Motivation for change: Implication for substance abuse. *Psychological Science, 10,* 209-213.

DiClemente, C.C. & Hughes, S. (1990). Stages of change profiles in outpatient alcoholism treatment. *Journal of Substance Abuse, 2,* 217-235.

DiClemente, C.C. & Porches, J.O. (1998). Toward a comprehensive transtheoretical model of change. In W.R. Miller & N. Heather (Eds.), *Treating addictive behaviors* (2nd ed.) (pp. 3-24). New York: Plenum.

Donovan, D.M. & Rosengren, D.B. (1999). Motivation for behavioral change and treatment among substance abusers. In J.A. Tucker, D.M. Donovan, & G.A. Marcatt (Eds.), *Changing addictive behavior* (pp. 127-159). New York: Guilford.

Greenstein, D.K., Franklin, M.E., & McGuffin, P. (1999). Measuring motivation to change: An example of the University of Rhode Island Change Assessment Questionnaire (URICA) in an adolescent sample. *Psychotherapy, 36*(1), 47-55.

Harris, G.A. (2001). Overcoming resistance with difficult clients. In B.K. Welo (Ed.), *Tough customers: Counseling unwilling clients* (2nd ed.). Lanham, MD: American Correctional Association.

Inciardi, J.A. (1994). *Screening and assessment for alcohol and other drug abuse among adults in the criminal justice system* (TIP 7). Rockville, MD: Center for Substance Abuse Treatment.

Jung, J. (2001). *Psychology of alcohol and other drugs.* Thousand Oaks, CA: Sage.

Kelman, H.C. (1971). Compliance, identification, and internalization: Three processes of attitude change. In B.C. Hinton & H.J. Reitz (Eds.), *Groups and organizations: Intergrated readings in the analysis of social behavior* (pp. 201-209). Belmont, CA: Wadsworth.

Lewis, J.A., Dana, R.Q., & Blevins, G.A. (1994). *Substance abuse counseling* (2nd ed.). Pacific Grove: Brooks/Cole.

McConnaughy, E., DiClemente, C., Prochaska, J.O., & Velicer, W. (1989). Stages of change in psychotherapy: A follow-up report. *Psychotherapy, 26,* 494-503.

McConnaughy, E., Prochaska, J.O., & Velicer, W. (1983). Stages of change in psychotherapy: Measurement and sample profiles. *Psychotherapy: Theory, Research and Practice, 20,* 368-375.

Miller, W.R. (1985). Motivation for treatment: A review with special emphasis on alcoholism. *Psychological Bulletin, 98*(1), 84-107.

Norman, G.J., Velicer, W.F., Fava, J.L., & Prochaska, J.O. (1998). Dynamic typology clustering within the stages for smoking cessation. *Addictive Behaviors, 23*(2), 139-153.

Palmer, J. (1994). The "effectiveness" issue today. In P.C. Kracoski (Ed.), *Correctional counseling and treatment* (3rd ed.) (pp. 15-30). Prospect Heights, IL: Waveland Press.

Platt, J.J., Buhringer, G., Kaplan, C.D., & Brown, B.S. (1998). The prospects and limitations of compulsory treatment for drug addiction. *Journal of Drug Issues, 18,* 505-525.

Prochaska, J.O., & DiClemente, C.C. (1986). Toward a comprehensive model of change. In W.R. Miller & N. Heather (Eds.), *Treating addictive behaviors: Processes of change* (pp. 3-27). New York: Plenum.

Prochaska, J.O., DiClemente, C.C., & Norcross, J.C. (1992). In search of how people change: Applications to addictive behaviors. *American Psychologist, 47,* 1102-1114.

Prochaska, J.O., Norcross, J.C., Fowler, J.L., & Follick, M.J. (1992). Attendance and outcome in a work site weight control program: Processes and stages of change as predictor variables. *Addictive Behaviors, 17*(1), 35-45.

Resnick, R.J. & Rozensky, R.H. (1996). *Health psychology through the life span: Practice and research opportunities.* Washington, DC: APA Press.

Romig, C. A. & Gruenke, C. (1991). The use of metaphor to overcome inmate resistance to mental health counseling. *Journal of Counseling and Development, 69*(May/June), 414.

Rosenthal, M.P. (1988). The constitutionality of involuntary civil commitment of opiate addicts. *Journal of Drug Issues, 18,* 641-662.

Rothfleisch, J. (1998). Comparison of two measures of stages of change among drug abusers. *Dissertation Abstracts International, 59,* 6-13. University Microfilm No. 0419-4217.

Rothschild, D. (1995). Working with addicts in private practice: Overcoming initial resistance. In A.M. Washton (Ed.), *Psychotherapy and substance abuse* (pp. 192-203). New York: Guilford.

Satel, S.L. (2000). Drug treatment: The case for coercion. In J. Tauber (Ed.), *National Drug Court Institute Review* (Vol. 3, No.1) (pp. 1-56). Alexandria, VA: National Drug Court Institute.

Serin, R. & Kennedy, S. (1997). *Treatment readiness and responsivity: Contributions to effective correctional programming.* Ottowa: Correctional Service of Canada, Research Branch.

Shearer, R.A. (1999). Resistance to counseling by offenders who abuse substances. *Annals of the American Psychotherapy Association, 2*(Sept./Oct.), 7.

Shearer, R.A. (2000). Coerced substance abuse counseling revisited. *Journal of Offender Rehabilitation, 30*(3/4), 153-171.

Shearer, R.A. (in press). Profiles of change: Adult male offenders in community correction residential treatment. *Corrections Management Quarterly.*

Shearer, R.A., Myers, L.B., & Ogan, G.D. (2001). Treatment resistance and ethnicity among female offenders in substance abuse treatment programs. *The Prison Journal, 81*(1), 55-72.

Shearer, R.A. & Ogan, G.D. (2002a). Measuring treatment resistence in offender counseling. *Journal of Addictions and Offender Counseling, 22*(2), 72-83.

Shearer, R.A. & Ogan, G.D. (2002b). Voluntary participation and treatment resistance in substance abuse treatment programs. *Journal of Offender Rehabilitation, 34*(3), 31-45.

Silverstein, M.E. (1997). The relationship among stages of change, attitudes towards treatment, and treatment investment in court-mandated outpatient substance abusers. *Dissertation Abstracts International, 57,* 10-13. University Microfilm No. 1419-4217.

Simourd, L. & O'Connor, T. (2000, June). Treatment readiness in a sample of probationers. Paper presented at the meeting of the Canadian Psychological Association, Ottawa, Ontario.

Stevens, P. & Smith, R.L. (2001). *Substance abuse counseling: Theory and practice* (2nd ed.). Upper Saddle River, NJ: Merrill Prentice Hall.

Velasquez, M.M., Maurer, G.G., Crouch, C., & DiClemente, C.C. (2001). *Group treatment for substance abuse.* New York: Guilford.

Velicer, W., Hughes, S., Fava, J., Prochaska, J., & DiClemente, C.C. (1995). An empirical typology of subjects within stages of change. *Addictive Behaviors, 20,* 299-320.

Vigdal, G.L. (1995). *Planning for alcohol and other drug abuse treatment for adults in the criminal justice system* (TIP 17). Rockville, MD: Center for Substance Abuse Treatment.

Walters, G.D. (2001). Overcoming resistance to abandoning a criminal lifestyle. In B.K. Welo (Ed.), *Tough customers: Counseling unwilling clients* (2nd ed.). Lanham, MD: American Correctional Association.

Willoughby, F.W. & Edens, J.F. (1996). Construct validity and predictive utility of the states of change scale for alcoholics. *Journal of Substance Abuse, 8*(3), 275-291.

Winick, B.J. (1997). *The right to refuse mental health treatment.* Washington, DC: American Psychological Association.

PART II:
INSTITUTIONAL-BASED
TREATMENT PROGRAMS

Under the rubric of rehabilitation, the history of treating inmates in adult prisons can be traced as far back as the first move toward incarceration as a tool of government. Meant to be more humane in nature, as we moved away from public floggings and some of our more corporal and often public forms of punishment, incarceration was primarily to be used as a time of penance for individuals thought to have been caught up in an unhealthy social milieu. It was believed that people could change given the proper instruction and that after a period of self-reflection and training they could be returned to society as law-abiding citizens. The medical model of corrections came out of this early thinking, and a variety of treatment programs found their way into America's prisons. Although it appeared for a time that the treatment approach to punishment might be a thing of the past, in recent years we have seen a return to our roots. The recognition of substance addiction as both a medical and social problem is certainly a step in that direction. The following chapters give examples of institutional-based treatment programs for inmates who are addicted to substances, complete with some of the problems associated with these treatment programs.

There is no doubt that the therapeutic community (TC) is the most highly recognized and used program of this type in the institutional setting (prisons and jails). In Chapters 4 and 5, the TC program within the Arkansas Department of Corrections is examined closely, with the two chapters using completely different methodological approaches. Golden, in Chapter 4, uses descriptive analysis of the clients within the Arkansas TC to point out some of the basic sociodemographic, criminal offense, drug abuse, and treatment characteristics of the clients and how those characteristics might be related to failure to complete the program. In Chapter 5, on the other hand, Patenaude uses a qualitative approach that consists of a series of focus groups with TC clients to explore their perspectives on this type of programming in the prison setting. Much of the chapter quotes exact comments from several clients and leaves the author questioning the efficacy of this type of treatment within the present context of the Arkansas prison system. Both Golden and Patenaude make recommendations to the Arkansas Department of Corrections in several areas, suggestions that could prove useful for correctional managers and administrators in other states as well.

In Chapter 6, Stohr et al. review findings from their study which asked inmates about their perceptions of a residential substance abuse treatment program, a program that takes place within the TC environment but with added components that come from a cognitive-behavioral approach. Based on their findings, they make several policy recommendations to administrators of already-existing programs, as well as to those correctional managers who are interested in beginning a program of this nature.

Chapter 4

A Critical Examination of Failures in a Therapeutic Community: Snatching Defeat from the Jaws of Victory

James W. Golden

In 1999, over 1.5 million drug arrests were reported by law enforcement agencies, accounting for an estimated 11 percent of the total arrests in the United States (FBI, 2000). In the state of Arkansas, there were 14,873 drug arrests which accounted for 6.8 percent of the total arrests for the year 2000 (Arkansas Crime Information Center [ACIC], 2001). Drug seizures nationwide increased dramatically between 1996 and 1999, with the confiscation of marijuana increasing from 1.4 million pounds to more than 2.3 million pounds, respectively. Cocaine seizures increased from 253,297 pounds in 1996 to 290,756 pounds in 1999 (Bureau of Justice Statistics [BJS], 2000a).

Approximately 61,000 prison inmates in 1998 reported that their offenses were committed in order to obtain money for the purchase of illegal drugs (BJS, 2000b). In addition, a study by the Bureau of Justice Statistics showed that 33 percent of state prisoners and 22 percent of federal prisoners committed their crimes while under the influence of drugs (BJS, 1999). A 1997 survey of state prison inmates indicated that 83 percent of them previously used marijuana, and 49 percent had used cocaine or cocaine-derived products. Approximately 20 percent reported using opiates, stimulants, hallucinogens, or depressants as well (BJS, 1997). Due to the consistent increases in the volume of drug-related crime and inmate drug history, many correctional institutions have seen fit to establish their own substance abuse treatment programs. Before the institution of drug treatment programs, addicts were consigned to mental health institutions or relegated to general prison populations to fend for themselves (Lester, Braswell, & Van Voorhis, 1992).

SUBSTANCE ABUSE TREATMENT
IN THE INSTITUTIONAL SETTING

In 1935, the same year Alcoholics Anonymous was founded (Lester et al., 1992), a research facility was established at the U.S. Public Health Service Hospital in Lexington, Kentucky. This unit would later be known as the Addiction Research Center. This center was the first to affiliate itself with a prison and offered treatment to addicted prisoners in a Lexington federal prison (National Institute on Drug Abuse [NIDA], 1995).

Substance abuse was regarded for some time after that as a physiological problem. It was not until the late 1960s that practitioners began to regard substance abuse and addiction as a psychological issue as well (Lester et al., 1992). In 1969, the National Institute of Mental Health (NIMH) established an agreement with Texas Christian University's Institute of Behavioral Research to design and implement a reporting system for drug abuse treatment programs. This program later became known as the Drug Abuse Reporting Program (DARP). The first two years of the program's existence were utilized for the collection of data for future research (Sells et al., 1974).

By 1979, 10,000 inmates were being served by 160 prison-based substance abuse treatment programs. This figure encompassed roughly 4 percent of the prison population in the United States. In 1989, the substance abuse treatment programs in U.S. prisons served 11 percent of the total inmate population (Chaiken, 1989).

During the 1980s, the substance abuse literature explored the characteristics of the client and how those attributes affect treatment success. Much of the recent research on prison substance abuse treatment programs, however, has focused on the attributes of the program, rather than the attributes of the client. This discussion attempts to refocus attention on client attributes by examining those inmates who were deemed failures and removed from a modified therapeutic community program at the Arkansas Department of Correction (ADC).

The ADC estimates that 83 percent of all inmates fit a profile indicative of substance abuse at intake. A little over half (55 percent) of all incoming inmates indicate a problem with alcohol, and 42 percent admitted using alcohol during the commission of their offenses. A large number of these inmates have been classified as frequent users. Inmates who report frequent drug use at the time of incarceration list their drug-of-choice preferences as alcohol, marijuana, and amphetamines. Most (66 percent) did not indicate participation in a substance abuse treatment program prior to incarceration.

The Arkansas Modified Therapeutic Community

The Arkansas Department of Correction has operated a substance abuse treatment program since 1980. The first program, using grant funds from the Arkansas Office of Alcohol and Drug Abuse Prevention, consisted of a thirty-day, twelve-step-oriented program that used inmates as peer counselors supervised by a correctional program manager. The SATP program graduated over 5,000 inmates in its first seven years of operation. Today, the program consists of fifteen different programs in thirteen units, including specialized programs at the boot camp and at the work-release centers. The ADC opened the Comprehensive Substance Abuse Treatment Modified Therapeutic Community in 1997. At inception, the program was six months long. It has been expanded to a nine-month program with beds for 120 participants at each of two different units.

Four goals have been identified by ADC for their therapeutic community. They include (1) building an intake program which effectively matches inmate needs with treatment programs; (2) creation of a comprehensive substance abuse treatment service using a therapeutic community model; (3) ensuring treatment gains continue after completion of the therapeutic community program; and (4) establishing a case coordination system that provides a community-based outreach service for individuals with substance abuse problems released from prison to the community.

The ADC therapeutic community utilizes a five-phase program. Phase 1 is a pretreatment orientation designed to introduce each client to the twelve-step program being used and to evaluate the inmate's degree of seriousness toward the program. Those who are willing to participate further move to Phase 2; those who are not serious about treatment are dropped. Phase 1 typically lasts for thirty days.

Phase 2 is focused on addressing the inmate's substance abuse and addiction issues along with faulty thinking associated with criminal behavior. A staff committee determines whether the inmate is ready for Phase 3, having met the goals and objectives of the inmate's comprehensive treatment plan and his or her overall program participation. This phase typically lasts for five months.

Phase 3 lasts a minimum of ninety days and is focused on relapse prevention, restructuring of the inmate's thinking processes, clarification of values, personality development, and positive cognitive restructuring. Educational and vocational issues are addressed, and prerelease counseling is conducted.

In Phase 4, the inmate begins prerelease continuing care to ensure treatment gains are maintained whether the inmate is still incarcerated or has been released on parole. If an inmate becomes parole eligible in Phase 3 or 4, the staff submits an aftercare plan to the Post Prison Transfer Board for their consideration prior to the inmate's release.

Phase 5 consists of continuing care in the community, which lasts up to twelve months following release from prison. Participants receive a full range of services based on needs and are monitored on a monthly basis by their respective parole officers and on a quarterly basis by the social worker/case coordinator from the therapeutic community.

The ADC modified therapeutic community is staffed with nine free-world staff members (three women and six men) and a correctional officer. Four of the staff are white and five are African American. In addition, there are thirteen inmate peer mentors or elders in the program. It borrows from examples of other jurisdictions such as Alabama, Florida, New York, and Wisconsin that run therapeutic community programs for substance abuse treatment (Tims, DeLeon, & Jainchill, 1994). Emulating these models, ADC houses treatment program participants separately from other inmates and maintains concentration on their substance abuse and related problems in a cooperative environment (see Patenaude & Laufersweiller-Dwyer, 2001). The ADC therapeutic community is a 120-bed unit located within the walls of the Tucker Unit, a male, maximum-security prison.

METHODOLOGY FOR THE PRESENT STUDY

Data for the present study were collected on 259 TC clients who were removed from treatment. This number represents 33 percent of the 812 admissions into the program since its inception. The sources of the data include client self-report measures and official data taken from the clients' files, including information collected during the intake process for the TC. The variables used in the study, as shown in Table 4.1, include demographic, social, offense, drug abuse, and treatment characteristics.

The overall purpose of the study was to discover possible predictors of failure in the ADC TC using the following four reasons for removal: (1) those who refuse treatment, (2) those who are noncompliant, (3) those who are therapeutic community rule violators, and (4) those who emphatically indicate that they want out of the program by breaking a unit or an ADC rule.

DATA ANALYSIS AND FINDINGS

A majority of the TC failures are Caucasian (59.8 percent) and 40.2 percent are African American. The mean age for these inmates is thirty-two, and over half of them reported being single (53.7 percent). The majority of inmates reported being a high school graduate or completing a GED certificate program (63.3 percent), with 13.9 percent reporting having some college. When using these variables to examine differences on reason for failure within demographic groups, no statistically significant differences were found. This means that race, age, marital status, and education levels were not found to be significant predictors of reason for failure.

Social Characteristics of TC Failures by Reason for Removal

We next examined the relationship between social characteristics of the inmate prior to entry into the TC and reason for failure. These include living status, family history of substance abuse, employment history, and disciplinary infractions earned since incarceration. Approximately one-quarter (26.6 percent) of inmates reported that they

TABLE 4.1. Variables used in the present study

Variable	Operationalization
Demographic characteristics	
Race	Race of the inmate
Age	Age of the inmate at entry into the system
Marital status	Marital status of the inmate at intake
Educational level	Education level at intake
Social characteristics	
Living status	Living status prior to incarceration
Family history	History of alcohol and/or drug abuse in the inmate's family
Employment history	Employment prior to incarceration
Disciplinary infractions	Number of disciplinary infractions while incarcerated
Offense characteristics	
Current offense	Primary offense/crime for which presently incarcerated
Arrest history	Number of times arrested in twelve months prior to present incarceration
Presence of violence at present offense	Offender currently serving time for a violent offense
Drug abuse characteristics	
First choice	Inmate's drug of choice
Treatment characteristics	
Time to removal	Time in days from entry to removal from program
Prior treatment	Previous substance abuse treatment

lived alone prior to incarceration, and 22.8 percent reported having lived with parents. Inmates who lived alone (30.1 percent) were more likely to violate a rule, refuse treatment (26.8 percent), and fail to comply (28 percent), while inmates who lived with parents (33.3 percent) were more likely to receive a disciplinary infraction that led to their removal from the program. The relationship between living arrangements and method of removal from the program was found to be statistically significant (χ^2 = 44.688, p < .018). Table 4.2 provides further detail on living arrangements and type of failure.

A little over half (56.4 percent) of the inmates failing the substance abuse treatment program report that they have a history of substance abuse in their family. Whites (65.1 percent) reported having a substance abuse history more often than did African Americans (34.9 percent), a relationship which is statistically significant (χ^2 = 3.799, p < .051). In terms of failure categories, those with a history of abuse refuse treatment 49.1 percent of the time, and those with no history of abuse refuse treatment 50.9 percent of the time. For noncompliance (56 percent), rule violation (62.7 percent), and disciplinary removals (56.4 percent), those reporting a history of abuse use in their family fail more often than their counterparts with no family substance abuse history, although the relationship between history of substance in the family is not statistically significant (χ^2 = 4.683, p < .197).

A majority of TC failures reported working full-time (62.5 percent) prior to incarceration. An additional 9.3 percent worked part-time, 1.2 percent were seasonal employees, 5.8 reported illegal employment such as drug sales, 10.4 percent were unemployed, 7.3 percent reported self-employment, and the remaining 3.5 percent reported other types of employment. Examining employment history and type of removal from the substance abuse program, those who were employed were removed for disciplinary reasons (76 percent) and noncompliance (72 percent) most often and for rule violations (62.7 percent) and refusal of treatment (55.4 percent) the least, but these differences are not statistically significant (χ^2 = 2.495, p < .869).

Next, we examined the number of disciplinary infractions recorded for inmates prior to entry into the program. Almost half (47.9 percent) recorded only a single disciplinary action. Inmates with more disciplinary infractions were more likely to be removed from the program for rule violations and disciplinary infractions. This relationship was found to be statistically significant (χ^2 = 107.796, p < .041).

These findings indicate that in terms of social characteristics, living status and the number of disciplinary infractions prior to admission into the TC have a greater effect on those who are removed from the program. Inmates who lived alone prior to incarceration and who

TABLE 4.2. Previous living arrangement and type of failure

Living arrangement	Refused treatment (%)	Noncompliance (%)	Rule violation (%)	ADC disciplinary (%)	Total (%)
Unknown	0.9	12.0	1.2	0.0	1.9
With spouse	8.9	4.0	8.4	2.6	7.3
With spouse and children	18.8	16.0	14.5	7.7	15.4
Alone	26.8	28.0	30.1	17.9	26.6
With parents	17.9	20.0	25.3	33.3	22.8
With other relatives	9.8	4.0	9.6	7.7	8.9
With friends	14.3	12.0	7.2	25.6	13.5
Institutionalized	0.0	0.0	1.2	2.6	0.8
Treatment facility	0.0	4.0	0.0	0.0	0.4
Homeless	2.7	0.0	2.4	2.6	2.3
Total	100.0	100.0	100.0	100.0	100.0

accumulated several disciplinary infractions were more likely to be removed from the TC.

Offense Characteristics of TC Failures by Reason for Removal

Almost half (48.6 percent) of the inmates in the present study reported no arrests in the twelve months prior to incarceration, 37.8 percent reported one arrest, and the remainder reported between three and seven arrests in the twelve-month period prior to incarceration. Of those reporting no arrests, 38.1 percent refused treatment, 13.5 percent were noncompliant, 31 percent were removed for a rule violation, and the remainder (17.5 percent) were removed for a disciplinary infraction, but these differences are not statistically significant.

Over half (52.5 percent) of treatment failures had been convicted of a violent offense. Of those removed for refusing treatment, 48.2 percent had been convicted of a violent offense. Those removed for noncompliance had the highest rate of conviction (60 percent) for a violent offense, followed by those with disciplinary infractions (59 percent) and those with rule violations (53 percent). There is, however, no statistically significant relationship between conviction of a violent offense and reason for treatment failure ($\chi^2 = 2.053, p < .561$).

Drug Abuse Characteristics of TC Failures by Reason for Removal

As shown in Table 4.3, the largest category for drug of choice is alcohol (30.1 percent), followed by marijuana or hashish (26.6 percent), amphetamines (18.5 percent), and none (10 percent). In addition, other drugs included heroin, other opiates, cocaine, tranquilizers, PCP, and crack cocaine. Alcohol (32.1 percent) is the leading drug of choice for those who refuse treatment. For those who are noncompliant, the leading drug of choice is none (28 percent) or alcohol (28 percent). Alcohol is also the drug of choice for those who leave the program for rule violations. For disciplinary infractions, however, the drug of choice becomes marijuana or hashish (38.5 percent). Further analyses, however, revealed that there is no statistically significant re-

TABLE 4.3. Drug of choice by reason for removal

Drug of choice	Refused treatment (%)	Noncompliance (%)	Rule violation (%)	ADC disciplinary (%)	Total (%)
None	5.4	28.0	13.3	5.1	10.0
Heroin	0.9	0.0	0.0	0.0	0.4
Other opiates/ synthetics	0.0	0.0	2.4	0.0	0.8
Alcohol	32.1	28.0	28.9	28.2	30.1
Amphetamines	23.2	12.0	16.9	12.8	18.5
Cocaine	2.7	4.0	6.0	5.1	4.2
Marijuana/hashish	27.7	24.0	20.5	38.5	26.6
Tranquilizers	0.9	0.0	0.0	0.0	0.4
Other	0.9	0.0	0.0	0.0	0.4
PCP	0.0	0.0	2.4	0.0	0.8
Crack cocaine	6.3	4.0	9.6	10.3	7.7
Totals	100.0	100.0	100.0	100.0	100.0

lationship between inmates' drug of choice and reasons for removal from the program ($\chi^2 = 33.839$, $p = < 287$).

Treatment Variables by Reason for Removal

Inmates in the ADC TC are subject to removal at any time during the program, with an average time to removal of eighty-five days. Of those who refused treatment (112, or 43.2 percent), the mean time to removal is seventy-five days, with half being removed within fifty-eight days. Twenty-five (9.6 percent) individuals were removed for noncompliance, and their time to removal averaged seventy-nine days. Eighty-three (32 percent) persons were removed from treatment for rule violations in an average of ninety-six days, and thirty-nine (15.2 percent) inmates were removed from treatment for disciplinary infractions with an average time of ninety days. Again, however, no statistically significant relationship was found between time to removal and reason for removal.

Over three-quarters (76.4 percent) of inmates removed from treatment have attended previous substance abuse treatment programs. This held true for those in the present study who refused treatment (76.8 percent), were found in noncompliance (72.0 percent), who violated rules (75.9 percent), or who received a disciplinary infraction (79.5 percent). The relationship, however, was not statistically significant ($\chi^2 = .496$, $p < .920$).

From a treatment standpoint, time to removal averages around eighty-five days, although the time ranges from as little as three days to 335 days. Those who have participated in some type of prior treatment program are more likely to refuse treatment or violate a rule to be removed from the ADC TC.

SUMMARY AND CONCLUSIONS

Pelissier et al. (1998) found that 12 percent of inmates in federal prisons either voluntarily drop out of programs or are removed for rule violations or disciplinary action. In Arkansas, and in the present study, that figure was 31.9 percent. Clearly, there is a need to examine reasons for why the ADC TC appears to be so much more unsuccessful at graduating clients from the program than those clients in federal

TCs. For the TC failures examined here, clients who had an unstable living arrangment or who lived alone or with their parents prior to incarceration were significantly more likely to fail to complete the program. Almost two-thirds (62.5 percent) of those failing the program were employed full-time prior to incarceration and were most often removed from the TC for disciplinary reasons (76 percent) or for noncompliance (72 percent). It appears that those who had a full-time job on the outside were having trouble adjusting to the social structure in prison.

The same can be said of those who report substance abuse problems in their family and those inmates who had accumulated a high number of ADC disciplinary infractions. Those TC failures who had previous substance abuse treatment were significantly more likely to refuse treatment or to violate a program rule in order to be removed from the TC.

In addition to these significant predictors of removal from the ADC TC, there are other possible explanations for failure. First is the requirement of the Post-Prison Transfer Board that all inmates who suffer from substance abuse complete the program prior to release from prison. Some inmates will start the process early, find the program not to be to their liking, and voluntarily remove themselves for one reason or another. They do so fully aware of the fact that they will have another opportunity to complete the program just prior to release. Second, in the ADC TC both alcohol and drug abusers are placed in the program for treatment. Although this joint program is necessary because of economic and staff restrictions, the programs should be separated so that more individualized and directed attention may be given to the often very different needs of these two types of substance abusers.

As noted by Patenaude and Laufersweiller-Dwyer (2001), the ADC TC program suffers from a great deal of inmate frustration and anger at being mandated into the program by what is perceived as coercive practices. Quite possibly, the mix of coerced and volunteer clients has contributed to the failure rate of the program. Unfortunately, the data do not provide clear distinctions between those who were mandated and those who volunteered. This may be due in part to inmates who, knowing how the system works, volunteer for the program knowing that the Post-Prison Transfer Board will require them to complete the program prior to release. Thus the inmate decides to have his "ticket punched" prior to the first appearance before the board.

Although this first look at reasons for failure in the ADC TC does provide correctional managers with a profile of those individuals who are more likely to be removed from treatment, a more in-depth analysis is called for. That step was taken by Patenaude through a qualitative study, utilizing a series of focus groups, in which current and former ADC TC clients were asked to give their perceptions of the program. The somewhat revealing and striking results of that study appear next in Chapter 5.

DISCUSSION QUESTIONS

1. Golden uses data from the same state correctional system as that used by Patenaude in Chapter 5 to describe issues associated with failure to complete Arkansas's institutional-based therapeutic community. How does Golden's approach to measuring the impact of this type of treatment differ from that used by Patenaude? Discuss any similarities related to overall findings between the two chapters.
2. What are some of the sociodemographic characteristics associated with failure to complete treatment in the inmate sample identified by Golden?
3. How would you describe the offense and drug abuse characteristics of program failures in the Arkansas prison therapeutic community?

REFERENCES

Arkansas Crime Information Center. (2001). *Crime in Arkansas 2000.* Little Rock: Statistical Analysis Center, Special Services Division.
Bureau of Justice Statistics. (1997). *Substance abuse and treatment, state and federal prisoners.* NCJ 172871. Available at <www.ojp.usdoj.gov/bjs>.
Bureau of Justice Statistics. (2000a). *Drug use, testing and treatment in jails.* NCJ 179999. Available at <www.ojp.usdoj.gov/bjs>.
Bureau of Justice Statistics. (2000b). *Sourcebook of criminal justice statistics.* NCJ 183727. Available at <www.ojp.usdoj.gov/bjs>.
Chaiken, M.R. (1989). *In-prison programs for drug-involved offenders.* Washington, DC: National Institute of Justice.

Federal Bureau of Investigation. (2000). *Crime in the United States*. Uniform Crime Reports. Available at <www.fbi.gov/ucr.htm>.

Lester, D., Braswell, M., & Van Voorhis, P. (1992). *Correctional counseling* (2nd ed.). Cincinnati, OH: Anderson Publishing Company.

National Institute on Drug Abuse. (1995). History of the addiction research center. *NIDA Notes, 10* (6).

Patenaude, A.L. & Laufersweiller-Dwyer, D.L. (2001). Arkansas Comprehensive Substance Abuse Treatment Program: Process evaluation of the Modified Therapeutic Community (Tucker Unit). Report Submitted to the Arkansas Department of Correction.

Pelissier, B., Wallace, S., O'Neil, J.A., Gaes, G.G., Camp, S., Rhodes, W., & Saylor, W. (1998). Federal prison residential drug treatment reduces substance use and arrests after release. Unpublished manuscript. Washington, DC: Federal Bureau of Prisons.

Sells, S. B., Joe, G.W., McRae, D.J., Simpson, D.D., Spiegel, D. K., Watson, D.D., & Watterson, O. (1974). *Research on patients, treatments and outcomes: Studies of the effectiveness of treatments for drug abuse,* Vol. 2. Cambridge, UK: Bellinger Publishing Company.

Tims, F.M., De Leon, G., & Jainchill, N. (1994). *Therapeutic community: Advances in research and application*. Washington, DC: National Institute on Drug Abuse.

Chapter 5

A Qualitative Exploration into a Prison Substance Abuse Treatment Program: "I Tell Them What They Want to Hear"

Allan L. Patenaude

The success of individual programming in institutional corrections begins with risk and needs assessments conducted during the reception and diagnostic phases and continues throughout an individual's sentence, with ongoing assessments of his or her progress in various treatment programs. Similar to substance abuse treatment programs that are offered to nonoffenders in the community, responsiveness to treatment is a primary concern in corrections, albeit one that is affected by the institutional environment and inmate culture.

The use of focus group interviews to understand the inmates' perceptions of the substance abuse treatment program delivered to inmates in a modified therapeutic community (TC) in an all-male prison is explored here. This discussion presents some of the difficulties, including access, honesty, confidentiality, compromise, etc., that are faced by researchers conducting qualitative research within correctional environments. Interestingly, while the literature on correctional programming has been quite vocal concerning the inmate's receptiveness for treatment as a factor in program success, few words have been written about the effects of the prison environment and inmate culture on the inmate's responsiveness during treatment. This discussion will also explore the effects of coerced treatment and offer insights into why inmates might be more likely than their free-world counterparts to reveal only what they believe the treatment staff and other inmates want to hear.

The site for this research was the Tucker Unit in the Arkansas Department of Correction (ADC). It is a nine-month, comprehensive program utilizing a modified therapeutic community mode of delivery. There is no separation of the inmate-clients based on their respective type of dependency (i.e., alcohol, cannabis, opiates, methamphetamines, etc.), as all participants receive the same recovery message. Nine months is considered the minimum duration for an inmate to successfully complete the TC program. All staff members have been certified as substance abuse counselors by the Arkansas Bureau of Alcohol and Drug Abuse Prevention (ADAP) and receive extensive, ongoing training throughout the year. The ranks of the treatment staff also include a small, yet significant, number of recovering addicts. In addition, the program receives inmate clients who have either volunteered to participate in the program or been mandated to complete it by the state's paroling authority, the Arkansas Post-Prison Transfer Board.

THERAPEUTIC COMMUNITIES IN PRISON ENVIRONMENTS

Pioneered by British physician Maxwell Jones at the end of World War II, therapeutic communities were designed as residential treatment regimes for patients with psychiatric disorders (Edwards, Arif, & Jaffe, 1983:148). Therapeutic communities would seek large-scale, social and psychological changes in their patients through activities which taught and promoted prosocial values. The general premise was that treatment staff could initiate these changes by empowering clients to contribute to their own therapy, and that of others, through a number of structured activities and the governance of the community. The formal structures and relationships found within most hospitals (i.e., downward from doctors through nurses to the patient or client) were replaced with more open communication and problem solving at the group level (Edwards et al., 1983).

The successes enjoyed by the British therapeutic communities did not go unnoticed by treatment professionals in the United States. In 1958, former addict Charles Dederich Sr. established the first American therapeutic community, Synanon, in Santa Barbara, California, to assist abusers of illegal drugs with their recovery (Yablonski, 1967). In marked contrast to the British TC model which employed a cooperative approach, Dederich instituted confrontational group sessions, such as the "Synanon Game," during which participants were empowered to say whatever they wanted to other members of the community.

Although Synanon's methods are controversial, the TC model has nonetheless been integrated into many community- and prison-based substance abuse treatment programs since the early 1970s including, for example, the U.S. penitentiary at Marion, Illinois, and Arizona's state prison at Fort Grant during 1969 (Lipton, Falkin, & Wexler, 1992:23). Therapeutic communities have been extremely successful in both environments.

The TC model has been modified for use within correctional settings since that time. Many states (including California, Florida, Texas, New York, Oregon, and Delaware) have developed residential programs based on a modified TC model within which the treatment program (1) is housed separately from the general prison population, (2) focuses on the inmate's substance abuse and related problems, and (3) lasts between six and twelve months (DeLeon, 1997; Lipton, 1997). Recognition of the value of this type of treatment intervention was given within the Violent Crime Control and Law Enforcement Act (1994) whereby the federal government created block funding to support those states who adopt "comprehensive approaches to substance abuse testing and treatment for offenders, including relapse prevention and aftercare services" (Violent Crime Control and Law Enforcement Act, 1994, HR 3355, Sec 1910[b]).

Florida's prison-based therapeutic communities may be held as the typical prison-based therapeutic community model and description, whereby:

> The TC treatment regimen uses self- and mutual-help approaches, peer pressure, and role-modeling in a structured environment to achieve the recovery goal. Peer pressure is seen as the catalyst that converts criticism and personal insight into positive change. High expectations and high commitment from both offenders and staff support this positive change. TCs provide a 24-hour-a-day learning experience in which individual changes in conduct, attitudes, and emotions are monitored and mutually reinforced in the daily regimen. . . . The goals of a residential TC include producing a change in lifestyle, abstinence from substance abuse, elimination of antisocial activity, increased employability, and prosocial attitudes and values. The

TC approach reinforces anticriminal modeling, promotes the understanding of social vs. didactic learning, and stresses the developmental process that occurs in a social learning context. (Bell, Mitchell, Bevino, Darabi, & Nimer, 1992:114-115)

Thus it is possible to see the dual legacies of Jones's original treatment philosophy and Dederich's Synanon-based approach intertwined within contemporary therapeutic communities.

One concern that arises within the treatment literature is the effectiveness and appropriateness of treatment when the client or patient is either forced by a judicial order to submit and complete a treatment program, or when his or her participation is the product of some other form of coercion such as the promise of early release from custody. Typical of the views on the inappropriateness of coerced or mandated treatment, for example, is that of addictions researcher Douglas Lipton (1998) who noted that

> [s]uccess in programs rarely occurs when the treatment is imposed on offenders in an authoritarian fashion, but is enhanced when the offenders are involved in developing their own program of recovery. This appears to be true whatever the form of treatment utilized. The program's intention should be to help prisoners help themselves rather than to "overhaul" them, cure them of their "illness," or "brainwash" them, or otherwise coerce a change of attitude. Forcing or compelling unwilling offenders to participate in programs (no matter how potent the program and how needful the inmate) should be avoided, since it is unlikely to generate much more than resentment, resistance and minimal change, or worse, faked change indicating apparent compliance. Involving *non-amenable* offenders is likewise unlikely to generate more than a minimal change in behavior, but fortunately it is likely not to foster counter effects. (Lipton, 1998:10)

Addictions researchers are, themselves, divided on the issue of coerced or forced treatment (cf. DeLeon, 1988; Gendreau, 1996; Harford, Ungerer, & Kinsella, 1976; Leukefeld & Tims, 1988). Their beliefs are polarized between those who hold that little benefit is realized from forced treatment of offenders who are not receptive to treatment and others who argue that few offenders will enter treatment without some form of external threat or motivation to do so. Unfortunately, for both researchers and practitioners, the jury remains undecided regarding the effectiveness of coerced treatment since there appear to be as many studies that point toward either the positive or negative aspects of coerced treatment as well as those studies which offer neutral or inconclusive findings (Anglin, Prendergast, & Farabee, 1998).

An additional problem may be found, according to Anglin et al. (1998), in the inconsistent terminology employed within the addictions and criminal justice fields concerning coerced treatment:

> "Coerced," "compulsory," "mandated," "involuntary," "legal pressure," and "criminal justice referral" are all used in the literature, sometimes interchangeably within the same article. This would not be a problem if these terms were synonymous. But "coercion" is not a well-defined entity; it in fact represents a range of options of varying degrees of severity across the various stages of criminal justice processing. "Coercion" can be used to refer to such actions as a probation officer's recommendation to enter treatment, a drug court judge's offer of a choice between treatment or jail, a judge's requirement that the offender enter treatment as a condition of probation, or a correctional policy of sending inmates involuntarily to a prison treatment program in order to fill the beds. In other cases, a treatment client's merely being "involved with the criminal justice system" is sufficient for him to be brought under the umbrella of "coercion." (Anglin et al., 1998:4-5)

In the Arkansas system, "coercion" is a practice that is both pervasive and as poorly defined as that presented by Anglin et al. (1998). Those Arkansas inmates with an alcohol- or drug-related offense who come before the Post-Prison Transfer Board are routinely mandated into the program as a condition for parole eligibility. This includes inmates who do not abuse drugs but who have been convicted of the manufacture, distribution, or sale of illicit alcohol or drugs. Both volunteer and mandated inmates participate in the same program.

QUALITATIVE RESEARCH
AMONG PRISON INMATES

Research within the field of corrections is rarely easy or uncomplicated. The three constituent groups—inmates, correctional staff, and administration—share a distrust for outside researchers since neither group can completely control what the latter will discover and report (Jackson, 1987; Jurik, 1985; Larivière & Robinson, 1996; Robinson, Simourd, & Porporino, 1991; Wright & Saylor, 1992). Qualitative researchers, in particular, are difficult to control since their major tools are observations and interviews (both individual and group).

Focus groups are a qualitative methodology that combine both observation and interviews. They employ first-person accounts of individual and group experiences on the analysis of conduct and social practices (Morgan, 1998; Vidich & Lyman, 1994). Focus group interviews, according to Morgan (1988:14), make "explicit use of the group interaction to produce data and insights that would be less accessible without the interaction found in a group."

Focus groups provide a qualitative methodology that is both exploratory and explanatory in nature. In the exploratory context, focus groups provide the opportunity to inquire into the range of issues that, other than those developed a priori to the research endeavor, are important to the participants. From the context of being explanatory research, focus groups offer researchers the opportunity to plumb the depths of the experiences as opposed to the prevalence of the conduct exposed by quantitative research. One additional strength of focus groups (and qualitative methods in general) is the flexibility that they provide. Should a new topic or issue emerge that has relevance to the research at hand, the focus group leader can shift efforts in that direction for however long is required.

Field researchers often face instant tests of credibility and personal integrity prior to and upon entering the field (see Patenaude, 2001; Patenaude & Laufersweiler-Dwyer, 2001). Among these challenges are the following interrelated issues:

1. *Gaining entry to the field:* Access may be granted or denied on the basis of whether senior managers perceive a value to the agency in the proposed research that outweighs any interruptions

of the normal prison routine caused by the research. In other words, what are operational or policy benefits of the research?

2. *Gaining and maintaining trust:* The field researcher must gain the trust of inmates, correctional staff, and managers alike in their first encounter. This requires assurances that what they reveal is important, that it will be reported in an accurate yet anonymous manner, and that it will not harm them or their respective positions in any manner. Here, perceptions of the research team as a neutral party are essential to gathering accurate information.

3. *Providing feedback:* Field researchers may be asked to provide an ongoing flow of research to the participants which is also a trust-based activity. This may take the form of brief summaries of what has been discovered during and between the numerous focus groups. Inmate participants will seek to understand what has been found and when the final research report will be available for their use, while program managers will require both regular updates and notification of serious problems as they are discovered; this is especially the case in process evaluations of specific treatment programs.

4. *Analysis and publication of the results:* Unlike quantitative researchers whose emphasis is the analysis and publication of aggregate data, the focus group facilitator gathers individual-level data and thus needs to ensure that his or her analysis guarantees the anonymity of the participants; for example, a statement accredited to an anonymous, black, female lieutenant when only two female lieutenants are employed in the unit is far from anonymous. Similarly, it is extremely easy and just as difficult for a field researcher to become biased toward individuals, small groups, or the populations of inmates, correctional staff, and managers.

Because of some of these obstacles, the research may be halted by the participants or the prison administration at any time should the researchers fail to meet essential challenges.

Shortly after the research for the present study was approved, for example, the program staff and the inmate hierarchy were given an approximation of the purpose of the research and how it would be conducted, and their respective cooperation was solicited. A small amount of anxiety was present during these initial meetings, with some members of the program staff exhibiting concern about the research. This concern produced attempts by the staff to delay the research by refusing entry into the unit to the researchers, to influence the researchers' perceptions of the program, to influence the conduct of the research through selective access, and to delay or restrict access to inmate program files and other program materials.

The impact of this type of interference by correctional staff to the research process can be handled, however, through intervention on the part of correctional managers. Managers made it clear to program staff the importance of the research and the need for cooperation in order to allow the researchers access to the data they would need in order to more accurately evaluate the program in question.

METHODOLOGY FOR THE PRESENT STUDY

A number of site visits were conducted throughout September 1999 and March 2001. Direct observation of daily activities permitted the researchers to explore that which Wholey (1994) termed the "entire program reality." The initial role of the evaluators was to observe the routine and minutiae of the daily program using known, nonparticipant observation techniques to understand the program activities, inmate participants, and program staff. This initial round of site visits provided the inmate population with an opportunity to become comfortable with the research team and project.

Later site visits required this role to change as it involved both semi-structured group interviews and focus groups to (1) understand participants' perspectives by understanding the particular context within which they act, (2) identify unanticipated phenomena, (3) understand the process by which events take place, (4) identify local causality, and (5) develop causal explanations (Geertz, 1973; Maxwell, 1992, 1996; Patton, 1990; Miles & Huberman, 1984). These interviews were held to gather client perceptions of the TC program and to provide a voice for their concerns in a manner which empowers them while protecting their identities (Marcus, 1994; Richardson, 1994). One interview involved only members of the inmate hierarchy, while the subsequent focus group interviews involved the remaining community members. Membership in the latter group interviews with current clients was nonexclusionary with the exception of the hierarchy members, who were excluded from the area in which the interviews were held. Finally, a session was conducted among program completers and noncompleters to explore the perceptions of persons who had nothing to gain or lose by talking with us.

The focus group interviews were facilitated by the author and handwritten notes were simultaneously taken by the two graduate students. This format permitted a more rapid exchange of ideas than could have occurred had the author been both facilitator and recorder of the proceedings. Tape recording was not regarded as an option in order to reinforce trust between the respondent and the researcher. The notes of the two graduate assistants were compared for accuracy.

For the purpose of this research, the generic phrases *staff member* and/or *program staff* were employed interchangeably to describe the free-world staff employed by ADC to operate the TC program. It provides anonymity and avoids otherwise unwieldy sentence structure. Similarly, although the terms *peer counselor, peer mentor, peer elder, expediter, department head,* and others were used interchangeably by the participants, both staff and inmate alike, they could be used to discern the identities of the persons involved. The terms *peer staff* and *inmate hierarchy* will be employed to offer a measure of protection to the respondents.

MAJOR FINDINGS

This section seeks to give voice to current and former participants in the ADC TC program. It does so primarily by way of the dialogic methodologies described earlier and the organization of the narrative itself.

Interviews with Peer Staff (Inmate Hierarchy)

Members of the inmate hierarchy comprised the first group interview. Throughout the interview, they repeated all of the comments one expects to hear from a sponsor in an Alcoholics Anonymous (AA) or Narcotics Anonymous (NA) meeting, or from a person about to graduate from a residential treatment program. Examples of these stock phrases are "This is one of the greatest things to happen to me," and "It has probably saved my life." Interestingly, the group tended to take its lead from two speakers who, as the other interviews would reveal, exercised both power and leadership in the program.

Despite the "party line" being provided to the evaluators, this group identified a number of areas for improvement of the program. The participants revealed that they perceived the orientation barracks process to be superior to the continuous, direct intake process that was being employed. "The old way," they said, "two guys met you at the door and you got caught up to speed real quick. Today, the setup is cyclical, and with clients in different stages of treatment throughout the program."

They also commented on the differences between the program participant who "volunteered" and the one who was "mandated" into the program by the Post-Prison Transfer Board (also referred to as the "Board," "Parole Board," or "PPTB") and the effects that the latter group has had on the overall TC program. They noted the following:

- Mandates reduce the number of volunteer slots open. We draw from other units and mandates get first dibs.
- They [mandates] make the process harder. Mandates are harder. They have a more "prove it to me" type of attitude. "I will prove you wrong."
- Don't have the parole board send them on a nine-month course when they only have six months of their sentence left. Half of the beds are filled by the parole board. By the time that we get him [a mandated inmate], he's back to the way he was before he was all nice to the parole board.

The structure of the program was also discussed by the hierarchy members. Many felt that the ADC policy of every inmate having a work assignment was interfering with the TC program. Two members noted:

- I don't like the way they split the day into a.m. and p.m. We went to four groups a day just to get chow time in. Some clients get a.m., some p.m.; this splits the community. There is also a confidentiality problem because of this and having to have an outside job. We are trying to build trust but someone outside is experimenting with us.
- It should be a eighteen-month program . . . maybe twelve months. . . . We could identify what's wrong in the first six months, have six months to plan a solution, and six months to implement it. We have to tinker to get things right. We don't

have a time frame, but we need a rules meeting every week, the same with criminal thinking sessions; there are some areas we could expand and others we could reduce.

Not only was the internal structure of the program discussed, but so too were external influences on the effective functioning of the program. One such external influence was the correctional staff assigned to the barracks. The choice of staff and their orientation toward the TC program were both viewed with concern as noted by the following comment:

- A definite set of officers would be good. There are some that do not need to be here, and it is difficult to confront their behavior. We need good, stable officers trying to reinforce what we are doing here.

Although the orientation of the individual correctional officer can, and does, have an influence on the smooth running of the program, these comments could also be interpreted as the inmate hierarchy claiming that "we have no control over" wanting to ensure that they remain the driving force in the therapeutic community and barracks. In summary, this group revealed a number of areas of improvement for the program. These areas included the following:

1. Differences between the program participant who "volunteered" and the one who was "mandated" into the program by the Post-Prison Transfer Board and the effects that the latter group has had on the overall TC program.
2. The current method of continuous, direct intake process, perceived as inferior to the previous orientation barracks process.
3. Problems caused in the TC program by the ADC policy that every inmate has a work assignment. This was seen as delaying the processes of change.
4. Difficulties caused by the lack of continuity and influence of correctional staff assigned to the barracks.

The inmate hierarchy has much to offer the therapeutic community. Indeed, they are essential to the effective operation of such a program whether it operates within or outside of a prison environment. However, care has to be taken to ensure that the hierarchy remains focused on the overall goal of the program. Some perspective was provided by one member of the current hierarchy who commented, "I'm in it for personal reasons as well as to help."

Interviews with Current Program Participants

The second set of five focus group interviews involved any current TC participant who was not a member of the inmate hierarchy. Although membership in the focus groups was somewhat fluid due to work assignments and counts, it remained constant at approximately twenty-five to thirty inmates per group. Willingness to participate in the group interviews and to honestly share experiences and concerns were the key criteria for including clients in this portion of the research. Similar to the previous interview with the inmate hierarchy, a number of themes emerged, including "this is a good program, but . . ."

The TC program is perceived by many participants as a good program, but one with a few structural problems. One inmate may have described it best as "the message is good, but there are problems with the messenger." Other comments included the following:

- This is my third time in the program. The first time I was pissed off by being mandated. The second time I tried, but it was hard. This time I am getting something out of it. After the previous times, I had taken a little of what I had learned here with me back out to the general population. I have now gotten a lot of educational stuff, like the "free your mind" class.

An issue related to the perceived positive components of the program is the delay or waiting period prior to admittance. Several inmates commented on this particular issue:

- There is a lot of good in the program, but it took me ten months to get in. Look around; there are ten empty beds today, but it took me almost a year to get in!
- I waited eight months to get in here. When I walked in there were eight empty beds.
- I was recommended by the parole board . . . that means mandated. It took me three months to get in. The parole board didn't

tell me I had to wait. There were empty beds in here! I want to know why? I could be out in January, but I still have four months of TC left.

This appears to be both a real and perceived concern because, on two occasions, the evaluators counted twelve and twenty empty beds, respectively, in one barracks alone. The issue of bed spaces versus waiting for an assignment to the TC is best comprehended, however, by taking the approach that (1) the TC at the Tucker Unit is an ADC-wide resource, (2) requests from both volunteer and board-mandated requests are difficult to coordinate and balance, and (3) the board-mandated inmates are a priority placement over volunteers.

The difference between inmates who volunteered and those who were mandated into the program remains an issue of contention. Many related that they felt coerced into taking the program. These concerns may be seen in the following comments:

- When I was at [another unit] I was mandated by the parole board. I had to sign a volunteer statement . . . I never volunteered; they made me sign a statement that I was volunteering to take this program or I couldn't be in it. It took me a year to get here so I signed it.
- I was mandated. I didn't sign a paper. Two months later I was in. You can sign the paper or do the time. They shipped me to the program.
- The board mandates you but makes you sign a form that you volunteer. Why mandate you if you have only a few months left to be in prison? They should mandate you early so you don't have to stay longer than if you were paroled.

Mandated inmates expressed both frustration and anger at what they perceived to be unfair practices by the Post-Prison Transfer Board. This anger was also directed at the TC program:

- They treat us like newborns. If they are mandated, a person should not be kicked out because they have a bad attitude. I volunteered. I didn't want to be mandated; that's a convict mentality. I could already have had it done if I were mandated. There are people who have been in the program for seven months and then been kicked out. I understand the chair [time out], but I can't understand how they can kick us out if they require us to do it.

- I am mandated. I was kicked out last year. It took me a whole year to get back in. That woman said when beds were open, people at the other units would have to respond, but the other units say they haven't heard from Tucker. [A program staff member] has good information, but I don't think I am getting anything out of it because I don't care. Because they are forcing me to listen to this. I don't want to quit, but I don't think the board should impose these kinds of stipulations on me.
- I'll be here for forty-five more days. My parole officer signed me up to do this. I am up on a ten-month parole violation, and I waited five months to get in.

As reported in the previous section, many of the inmates in the current TC inmate population regard the program favorably, but the "messengers," the sanctions court, and the inmate hierarchy received less than positive comments. Regarding the inmate hierarchy, several current clients expressed the following frustrations:

- I have seen people kicked out [by the inmate hierarchy] for bullshit reasons. Sometimes the peer mentors make up rules as they go along.
- One thing I don't understand is placing one convict over another convict. It is a bunch of criminals picking at each other and we're being taught by [inmates who have committed serious crimes]. I can't look past that.
- I don't like the inmate police. You have to be a rat or a snitch. Somebody is going to do something horrible.

A large amount of hostility was directed toward the sanctions imposed by both the program staff and the inmate hierarchy in the sanctions court. Most of the frustration appears to be related to being ordered to engage in certain embarrassing behavior (sitting in chairs facing the wall all day) by fellow inmates. Further, inmates expressed concern about their sworn statements, or those of witnesses brought before the court to speak on behalf of the inmate, as not being "worth much."

In summary, the interviews with current TC clients revealed that most inmates perceived the program as a "good program" but one not

without problems. Clients perceived a great deal of difference between those clients who were mandated to treatment and those who
volunteered. Mandated clients expressed anger and frustration about
"unfair" practices by the Post-Prison Transfer Board, especially
when it comes to having to wait for entry into the program. Clients
were also concerned about some of the program staff not "buying
into" the TC community and with breaches in confidentiality by program participants as they journeyed beyond the TC environment to
individual work assignments in other parts of the prison. Finally, a
great deal of hostility was expressed toward the TC sanctions court
and the sanctions imposed by both the program staff and the inmate
hierarchy.

Former TC Clients

A semi-structured, group interview of former clients was next conducted, with no attempt made to discriminate on the basis of success
or failure in the program. The former clients expressed an extremely
high level of frustration and anger toward both current and former TC
participants. The members of the inmate hierarchy were the primary
targets of this hostility, followed by the sanctions court, the program
staff, and the mixing of volunteers and mandated inmates, respectively.

According to former TC clients, the inmate hierarchy is best described as a power elite with its members' interests being the fore-
most consideration. Many felt that the actions of the inmate hierarchy
are sanctioned by the program staff. Several inmates commented on
this issue:

- They ain't doing nothing right. One inmate has control over another. Brother [hierarchy member] is like a cop. He'll turn any-
  body in on anything. He's a convict just like we are!
- Brother [hierarchy member] intimidates TC clients . . . free-
  world staff give him enough power to terminate inmates.
- I did six months in there and made them kick me out. Lot of sick
  individuals are placed in peer mentoring positions!
- Inmates shouldn't be over other inmates. They don't want you to
  succeed.
- So much bullshit around you . . . so much shit goin' on down.
  You can't concentrate on the good. They force you to snitch and

> if you don't they snitch on you for not doing it . . . gets you so stressed.
>
> • There are peer counselors who are sexual offenders. That is not supposed to happen. How can they tell me how to run my life?

Inconsistency and favoritism on the part of the hierarchy members of the sanctions court, accompanied by acquiescence on the part of the program staff to the inmate hierarchy, were the most common negative responses. Much of this frustration was similar to that expressed by current TC clients, as demonstrated by the following comments:

> • They make you wear signs like "jackass." This gives you low self-esteem. Inmates having authority over you is not right.
> • It [sanctions court] occurs on Sundays and no free-world staff are around then. There is no defending yourself.

The TC program staff were the next major targets of this particular group's anger. As was found with the current TC clients, it was generally believed that the information provided in the program is useful. The real or perceived treatment of the program staff and the inmate hierarchy, however, greatly reduces any positive impact of the program.

Overall, the former TC clients had similar suggestions as did the current clients when it comes to improving the ADC TC. Again, one of the most common suggestions concerned the separation of volunteers and mandated inmates into two separate TC programs, followed by the suggestion that the inmate peer mentoring system be removed from the program altogether. This group of inmates also suggested a restructuring of the sanctions court, with more input about how it should be conducted coming from the clients themselves.

HONESTY WITHIN TREATMENT PROGRAMS

The issue of honesty in group and individual counseling was explored, based in part on the comments about inmates having control over other inmates and perceptions of differential handling of clients by program staff. The question posed here was "How truthful or hon-

est can you be in group sessions?" This question was usually followed by loud laughter and comments such as these:

- I can't be that honest!
- If I tell them the truth it will be down the hall [into other bar-
  racks]. Confidentiality is shit!
- I am truthful and honest. I just hold stuff back. I hold back per-
  sonal stuff like my addiction . . . like why I was doing things.
  What I say is the truth just, most of it, doesn't come out.
- Some things I don't say. It's not like seeing a psychiatrist.
  Here, I will tell them only what the f**ck they want to hear and
  go on. . . . I tell them what I have to tell them so I can go home.

Honesty within treatment programs is seen to be a major indicator
of treatment responsiveness. Lipton (1998; Lipton et al., 1992) identified this concern among coerced participants in free-world and correctional treatment programs whom he believed might fake change to
indicate apparent compliance with the program and its objectives.
The inability to be honest in the program does not appear to be a major concern to these inmates, but it should be a concern of the
program staff and ADC management.

Lipton (1998:10) argued that inmates could be enticed into programs that encourage participation by "making staying in the program
more desirable than leaving. They do this by creating an environment
that is physically safer, cleaner, and more secure psychologically than alternative custodial environments." What Lipton (1998) and others have
neglected to explore, however, is the effect that the environment of the
prison has on the inmate's ability to be honest with other inmates in the
program. In a program such as the one described here, in which inmates are required to spend lengthy periods of time working outside
the treatment barracks among other inmates, the ability to create an environment that is psychologically secure is nearly impossible.

SUMMARY AND CONCLUSIONS

The Comprehensive Substance Abuse Treatment Program (CSATP)
operating as a modified therapeutic community within the ADC
meets most of the general criteria for effective therapeutic communi-

ties in both the free-world and correctional environments. Few substantive areas need to be modified. Participants' perceptions account for the majority of concerns.

Inmate participants have difficulty identifying with this TC program and feel a general need for improvement in the program. Time spent in the program did not appear to have an effect in this area. Not only did a large number of inmates not feel that they are part of the program, they also did not perceive the program staff to be members of the TC community. Rather, they were viewed as members at a distance with specific roles.

A number of specific policy changes have been recommended to ADC as the result of this study. Among these recommendations were the following:

1. modify the influence of the community hierarchy and the operation of the sanctions court;
2. change the participant selection process;
3. increase staffing levels and revise staffing patterns;
4. increase consistency in the application of rules;
5. change volunteer-mandate ratio;
6. increase aftercare provisions for clients;
7. develop a method to discuss and evaluate honesty within the program; and
8. continue monitoring the CSATP and gather data for an outcome evaluation.

This study has illustrated the benefits of including qualitative methods as part of most, if not all, correctional research involving inmates or staff. It is believed that correctional managers and treatment staff would have identified the concerns noted herein through the use of quantitative methods such as survey questionnaires and file data, but the nature of the problems and possible ways to correct them is best gathered though interaction with and among the persons being studied.

DISCUSSION QUESTIONS

1. How would you describe the major goals and objectives of the therapeutic community?

2. As identified by Patenaude through a series of focus groups with Arkansas prison inmates, discuss problems associated with that particular institutional-based therapeutic community.
3. What point do you think Patenaude is making with his use of the subtitle "I Tell Them What They Want to Hear"? What are the implications here for correctional managers and treatment providers?

REFERENCES

Anglin, M.D., Prendergast, M., & Farabee, D. (1998). The effectiveness of coerced treatment for drug-abusing offenders. Paper presented at the Office of National Drug Control Policy's Conference of Scholars and Policy Makers, Washington, DC, March 23-25.

Bell, W.C., Mitchell, J.G, Bevino, J., Darabi, A., & Nimer, R. (1992). Florida department of corrections' substance abuse programs. In C.G. Leukefeld & F.M. Tims (Eds.), *Drug abuse treatment in prisons and jails* (pp. 110-125). Washington, DC: National Institute on Drug Abuse, U.S. Department of Health and Human Services.

DeLeon, G. (1988). Legal pressure in therapeutic communities. In C.G. Leukefeld & F.M. Tims (Eds.), *Compulsory treatment of drug abuse: Research and clinical practice* (pp. 236-249). Washington, DC: National Institute on Drug Abuse, U.S. Department of Health and Human Services.

DeLeon, G. (1997). Modified therapeutic communities: Emerging issues. In G. DeLeon (Ed.), *Community as method: Therapeutic communities for special populations and special settings* (pp. 261-270). Westport, CT: Greenwood Publishing.

Edwards, G., Arif, A., & Jaffe, J. (Eds.). (1983). *Drug use and misuse: Cultural perspectives based on a collaborative study by the World Health Organization.* London: Croom Helm.

Geertz, C. (1973). *The interpretation of cultures.* New York: Basic Books.

Gendreau, P. (1996). The principles of effective intervention with offenders. In A.T. Harland (Ed.), *Choosing correctional options that work: Defining the demand and evaluating the supply* (pp. 117-130). Thousand Oaks, CA: Sage Publishing.

Harford, R.J., Ungerer, J.C., & Kinsella, J.K. (1976). Effects of legal pressure on prognosis for treatment of drug dependence. *American Journal of Psychiatry, 133*(12), 1399-1403.

Jackson, B. (1987). *Fieldwork.* Urbana: University of Illinois Press.

Jurik, N.C. (1985). Individual and organizational determinants of correctional officer attitudes towards inmates. *Criminology, 23*(3), 523-539.

Larivière, M. & Robinson, D. (1996, February). *Attitudes of federal correctional officers towards offenders.* Ottawa, Ontario: Correctional Service of Canada. Available at <http://www.csc-scc.gc.ca/>.

Leukefeld, C.G. & Tims, F.M. (1988). Compulsory treatment: A review of findings. In C.G. Leukefeld & F.M. Tims (Eds.), *Compulsory treatment of drug abuse: Research and clinical practice* (pp. 236-251). Washington, DC: National Institute on Drug Abuse, U.S. Department of Health and Human Services.

Lipton, D.S. (1997). *The effectiveness of treatment for drug abusers under criminal justice sanction.* Washington, DC: National Institute of Justice.

Lipton, D.S. (1998). Principles of correctional therapeutic community treatment programming for drug abusers. Paper presented at the ONDCP Consensus Meeting on Treatment in the Criminal Justice System, Washington, DC, March 25.

Lipton, D.S., Falkin, G.P., & Wexler, H.K. (1992). Correctional drug abuse treatment in the United States: An overview. In C.G. Leukefeld & F.M. Tims (Eds.), *Drug abuse treatment in prisons and jails* (pp. 8-30). Washington, DC: National Institute on Drug Abuse, U.S. Department of Health and Human Services.

Marcus, G.E. (1994). What comes (just) after "post"? The case of ethnography. In N.K. Denzin & Y.S. Lincoln (Eds.), *Handbook of qualitative research* (pp. 563-574). Thousand Oaks, CA: Sage Publications.

Maxwell, J.A. (1992). Understanding and validity in qualitative research. *Harvard Educational Review, 62*(2), 279-300

Maxwell, J.A. (1996). *Qualitative research design: An interactive approach.* Thousand Oaks, CA: Sage Publishing.

Miles, M.B. & Huberman, A.M. (1984). *Qualitative data analysis: A sourcebook of new methods.* Beverly Hills, CA: Sage Publications.

Morgan, D.L. (1988). *Focus groups as qualitative research.* Newbury Park, CA: Sage Publications.

Patenaude, A.L. (2001). Analysis of issues affecting correctional officer retention within the Arkansas Department of Correction. *Correction Management Quarterly, 5*(2), 49-67.

Patenaude, A.L. & Laufersweiler-Dwyer, D. (2001). *Arkansas Comprehensive Substance Abuse Treatment Program: Process evaluation of the Modified Therapeutic Community (Tucker Unit).* Washington, DC: National Institute of Justice.

Patton, M.Q. (1990). *Qualitative evaluation and research methods* (2nd ed.). Newbury Park, CA: Sage Publishing.

Richardson, L. (1994). Writing: A method of inquiry. In N.K. Denzin & Y.S. Lincoln (Eds.), *Handbook of qualitative research* (pp. 516-529). Thousand Oaks, CA: Sage Publications.

Robinson, D., Simourd, L., & Porporino, F.J. (1990). *Research on staff commitment: A discussion paper.* Ottawa, Ontario: Correctional Service of Canada. Available at <http://www.csc-scc.gc.ca/>.

Vidich, A. & Lyman, S. (1994). Qualitative methods: Their history in sociology and anthropology. In N.K. Denzin & Y.S. Lincoln (Eds.), *Handbook of qualitative research* (pp. 23-59). Thousand Oaks, CA: Sage Publications.

Wholey, J.S. (1994). Assessing the feasibility and likely usefulness of evaluation. In J.S. Wholey, H.P. Hatry, & K.E. Newcomer (Eds.), *Handbook in practical program evaluation* (pp. 15-39). San Francisco: Jossey-Bass.

Wright, K.N. & Saylor, W.G. (1992). A comparison of perceptions of the work environment between minority and non-minority employees of the federal prison system. *Journal of Criminal Justice, 20,* 63-71.

Yablonski, L. (1967). *Synanon: The tunnel back.* Baltimore, MD: Penguin Books.

Chapter 6

Residential Substance Abuse Treatment Programming: What Do the Inmates Think?

Mary K. Stohr
Craig Hemmens
Jed Dayley
Diane Baune
Kristin Kjaer
Mark Gornik
Cindy Noon

Drug and alcohol use and abuse are responsible for many social ills, not the least of which is an association with criminal involvement (Associated Press 1998; National Center on Addiction and Substance Abuse [CASA], 1998). According to a recent Bureau of Justice Statistics (BJS) report, nationally about 47 percent of probationers, 60 percent of jail inmates, and 49 percent of state prison inmates were under the influence of drugs or alcohol at the time of their arrest or commission of their crime (Associated Press, 1998). The authors of a report released by the National Center on Addiction and Substance Abuse at Columbia University revealed that "[d]rug and alcohol abuse and addiction are implicated in the incarceration of 80%—1.4 million—of the 1.7 million men and women behind bars today" (CASA, 1998). Idaho inmates are similarly afflicted with alcohol and

This chapter is a modified version of Stohr, M.K., Hemmens, C., Kjaer, K., Gornik, M., Dayley, J., Noon, C., & Baune D. (2002). Inmate perceptions of residential substance abuse treatment programming. *Journal of Offender Rehabilitation,* 34(4), 1-32. Reprinted with permission of The Haworth Press, Inc.

drug use problems. Between 1993 and 1994, 1,139 inmates were surveyed at the Reception and Diagnostic Unit in the Idaho Department of Corrections (IDOC). Among these offenders, 23.7 percent had been using drugs, 43.3 percent had been using alcohol, and 10.1 percent had been using both at the time of the commission of their offense (Cardenas, 1996).

The treatment program studied here is set in a therapeutic community. Therapeutic communities (or TCs) have been used to treat a variety of disorders, including substance abuse (Farabee, Prendergast, & Anglin, 1998; Finney, Moos, & Chan, 1981; Hartmann, Wolk, Johnston, & Colyer, 1997) and mental illness (McMurran, Egan, & Ahmadi, 1998). The TC method of treating substance abuse involves a combination of social and psychological therapy designed to alter the client's attitudes, beliefs, and behavior. The treatment occurs in a group setting, and peer interaction is a major component of the process. Personal responsibility and mutual assistance are emphasized (Corrections Alert, 1998).

Therapeutic communities have been much studied, and reviews of the literature indicate the TC model holds promise for reducing substance abuse and recidivism among drug-using inmates (Hartmann et al., 1997; Knight, Simpson, & Hiller, 1999; Lipton, 1998; Lockwood, McCorkel, & Inciardi, 1998; Martin, Butzin, Saum, & Inciardi, 1999; Pearson & Lipton, 1999; Wexler, 1995; Wexler, Melnick, Lowe, & Peters, 1999). Although therapeutic communities were originally designed for free-world settings, there has been a recent increase in the implementation of TCs in institutional settings, particularly corrections (see generally, Cullen, Jones, & Woodward, 1997; Early, 1996).

The Residential Substance Abuse Treatment (RSAT) program at the South Idaho Correctional Institution (SICI), which began accepting inmate clients in May 1997, is designed to fill a need for substance abuse treatment among the Idaho correctional population. The program targets reincarcerated parole violators with substance abuse problems. Idaho Department of Correction data indicate that the majority of such offenders have alcohol or methamphetamine dependencies. The RSAT program design includes an intensive nine- to twelve-month treatment regimen for chronic substance abusers which addresses both addiction and criminality in a structured therapeutic environment, based on the TC model. In addition, the Idaho Parole Commission and the IDOC have engaged in a cooperative arrangement whereby successful completion of the program will likely result in the inmate receiving a parole date.

An important and distinguishing feature of the RSAT plan is the use of a combination of treatment modalities, including cognitive self-change and twelve-step programming, in a curriculum that is divided into a series of three-month phases. There is a focus on identifying thinking and behaviors—via group process, thinking reports, and journal writing—which place the participant at risk of a relapse to substance abuse and/or criminal behavior. These activities all take place within the parameters of a therapeutic environment in a dedicated tier of the SICI (Cardenas, 1996; State of Idaho, 1998).

Study of such a mixed-modality program that integrates the cognitive and behavioral pieces and aftercare with the more traditional twelve-step and TC components is exciting. This is particularly so because of the emerging evaluation literature that supports the importance of addressing cognition, reinforcing the positive over the negative behaviors (and client involvement in this) and follow-through in treatment upon release (Andrews et al., 1990; Antonowicz & Ross, 1997; Gendreau & Ross, 1987, 1995; Henning & Frueh, 1996; Husband & Platt, 1993; Inciardi, 1995; McMurran, 1995).

While the efficacy of prison-based therapeutic communities has received much attention in the research literature (Hiller, Knight, Broome, & Simpson, 1998; Knight, Simpson, Chatham, & Camacho, 1997; Lipton, 1998; Rouse, 1991), and some attention has been paid to the individual treatment components (Farabee et al., 1999; Gendreau & Ross, 1995; Hartmann et al., 1997; Incorvaia & Kirby, 1997; Wexler & Williams, 1986), very little attention has been paid to the attitudes and perceptions of the inmate clients. In an effort to fill this gap in the literature, and as part of an NIJ-funded process evaluation of the Idaho RSAT program, we examined the attitudes and perceptions of the Idaho RSAT inmates. In this chapter we report the results of our research.

RESEARCH ON CORRECTIONAL PROGRAMMING

The literature on substance abuse and related programming is replete with research evaluations that indicate successful treatment programming can be designed and implemented in the correctional environment (Andrews et al., 1990; Bowman, Lowrey, & Purser, 1997; Calco-Gray, 1993; Farabee et al., 1999; Field, 1985, 1992; Gendreau & Ross, 1995; Hartmann et al., 1997; Henning & Frueh, 1996; Inciardi, 1995; Lipton, 1998; Lipton, Falkin, & Wexler, 1992; Office of Justice Programs, 1998; McMurran, 1995; Palmer, 1995; Rice & Remy, 1998).The most successful programs are those that combine the delivery of substantive knowledge in an environment that is suited to therapeutic change (Inciardi, 1995; Lipton et al., 1992). Research also indicates that cognitive attributes, positive modeling, behavioral redirection, emotional therapy, a treatment environment engendering trust and empathy, and intensive involvement in problem solving by clients in their own treatment are also key to attaining actual behavioral change upon release (Andrews et al., 1990; Antonowicz & Ross, 1997; Gendreau & Ross, 1987, 1995; Henning & Frueh, 1996; Inciardi, 1995; McMurran, 1995; Pollock, 1997; Smith & Faubert, 1990). Treatment programs directed at drug offenders also appear to achieve greater success in reducing recidivism when services were continued postrelease (Hanlon, Nurco, Bateman, & O'Grady, 1999; Lipton, 1998; McMurran, 1995; Rouse, 1991; Siegal et al., 1999; Tims & Leukefeld, 1992; Wexler, DeLeon, Thomas, Kressel, & Peters, 1999).

The three therapeutic communities located in the Delaware Correctional System and as described by Inciardi (1995) incorporated a number of the attributes that appear to be related to more successful programming in correctional environments. These programs combined behavioral, cognitive, and emotional therapies, as well as other techniques, in treatment regimens designed to address individual needs of the substance-abusing clientele. Significantly, after six months the clients who had participated in treatment were more likely to be drug and arrest free than the comparison group (Inciardi, 1995). At eighteen months, those who had completed the program were three times more likely to be drug free than those who had not completed the program (Office of Justice Programs, 1998).

Henning and Frueh (1996) reported that a cognitive-behavioral treatment model program in a Vermont medium-security prison achieved some success in the reduction of recidivism by participants relative to a comparison group. After acknowledging some limitations to their study, they report a "29% reduction in the recidivism rate of the treatment group compared to the no-treatment group" (Henning & Frueh, 1996:537).

Of course, the promise of correctional programming has not always been realized. In the widely cited and influential review of correctional programming by Martinson (1974) and Lipton, Martinson, & Wilks (1975), it was revealed that not much has worked to reduce the recidivism rate of participants. More recent meta-analyses of correctional programming (e.g., Antonowicz & Ross, 1997; Leukefeld & Tims, 1992; Logan & Gaes, 1993; Wright, 1995) have also raised serious questions concerning the veracity of claims of success by correctional program proponents. As Antonowicz and Ross (1997:313) indicate, after reviewing the published research on correctional programming from 1970 to 1991:

> There is not a large number of published, rigorously controlled studies. Many published studies have either inadequate control/comparison groups, do not report on sample size, use sample sizes that are too small to enable statistical tests, or fail to examine outcome.

Moreover, of the forty-four programs that had adequate research designs, they found that only twenty were effective (Antonowicz & Ross, 1997). Those programs that achieved some success in their and others' meta-analyses (e.g., see Andrews et al., 1990; McMurran, 1995) were stronger in the areas of conceptualization (programs with cognitive-behavioral models, structuring, and role-playing). They included a greater variety of programming options and techniques, targeted factors that were actually related to criminal involvement, and matched offender learning styles to complementary services.

Programs also falter because of external factors. Leukefeld and Tims (1992), in the introduction to their edited monograph on the state of substance abuse programming in corrections, caution that programs must be given time to succeed or fail on their merits. By this they mean that in order to succeed, programs must have sustained adequate funding over a period of time and must be designed with evaluation in mind. Such a design should be realistic in scope and time line with respect to outcomes and subject participation (Leukefeld & Tims, 1992; Schuiteman & Bogle, 1996). Similarly, Lipton et al. (1992) found in their review of evaluations of two well-studied correctional therapeutic community substance abuse programs, the New York "Stay'n Out" and the Oregon "Cornerstone" programs, that recidivism in crime and substance use decreased for participants as compared to control groups. They note, however, that the history of therapeutic community program demise over the past two decades is often tied to factors external to those programs such as administrative changes and funding reductions.

Although the majority of the research on prison therapeutic communities is focused on description of the program components or outcome evaluation, several researchers have examined an understudied aspect of the process—the attitudes and perceptions of the program participants. Lemieux (1998) examined the influence of a variety of inmate characteristics on their perceptions of their postrelease adjustment and found that social support was a significant factor. McCorkel, Harrison, and Inciardi (1998) compared the perceptions of program completers and dropouts and found that those who left the program viewed it more as punishment than treatment. In this chapter we expand upon this limited research on inmate/client perceptions, focusing on the perceptions of the RSAT program among current Idaho RSAT inmates. Given that the success of therapeutic communities hinges on the meaningful involvement and decision making of their clients, the perceptions of program efficacy by those clients should be a key component of a process evaluation.

RSAT AT SICI

The SICI therapeutic community treatment program was designed to achieve reduced recidivism of substance-abusing offenders and collaterally to decrease the costs of crime and reincarceration for victims and taxpayers. RSAT was designed as a therapeutic community within a prison setting, and it employs cognitive self-change and behavioral strategies.

Treatment Components

The *therapeutic community* is "a residential-based, substance abuse treatment modality incorporating the use of a social learning model based on peer support for pro-social values and behaviors" (Hartmann et al., 1997:18). A key aspect of the TC is a recognition that a community can provide an individual with the strength, support, and insight to make needed changes that would be much more difficult if that person were on his or her own.

> In this TC setting each individual has the opportunity to grow, as a community member, in ways not possible by going it alone. A community environment also allows its members to fight a common enemy and reach a common goal. In the RSAT program the common enemy is an addictive and criminal lifestyle. The common goal is personal change by learning new ways of "Right Living." (CompCare, 1998:4)

Social learning theories provide the framework for effective cognitive-behavioral approaches to treatment (Gendreau, 1993; National Institute of Corrections [NIC], 1997). *Cognitive self-change* and *behavioral strategies* are utilized in this program to provide inmates with the ability to consider the thinking errors that lead to substance use/abuse and to provide them with the means to move down an alternate and less self-destructive path (NIC, 1997). Key concepts of this treatment method include cognition and modeling. There is a recognition of both the connection between "[t]he person (cognitive thought processes or awareness), the behavior and the environment" (NIC, 1997:12) and the importance of learning through positive modeling.

The SICI RSAT program employs the following strategies to achieve a change in thinking and behavior: group process, thinking reports, and journals. The group process is initially focused on providing clients with information so that they might better understand the connection between thinking and behavior. Next, the group focuses on individual identification of thinking errors and practicing interventions over a period of time so that these interventions might become part of alternate and more prosocial thought processes. The group process is structured by five guidelines: depersonalized staff authority that maintains control and adherence to rules; allowing the individual offender to be the authority on issues related to how they think and how they should think; focus on the basic steps of cognitive change; work to achieve cooperation between group members and staff; and involvement of all group members in the process (Boise CareUnit, 1997).

Thinking reports are used by individuals to objectively identify specific thoughts and feelings associated with high-risk behavior in a given situation. Journals are used to document the process that the individual is involved in thinking about and then reevaluating their behaviors and motivations. In addition, both the thinking reports and the journals are to be regularly reviewed by staff and inmates as a means of measuring progress in treatment.

Inclusion of the Minnesota Model of Chemical Dependency (twelve-step program) is central to this RSAT regimen. The components of the program include the use of group and the use of recovering alcoholics/addicts as counselors. The program also utilizes individual counseling with professional staff, lectures, group reading, life history work, Alcoholics Anonymous (AA) and/or Narcotics Anonymous (NA) attendance, twelve-step work, and recreational and physical activity (Boise CareUnit, 1997:54). The four key elements of the Minnesota Model that are emphasized in the RSAT program are as follows:

1. A belief that addicts can change their beliefs, attitudes, and behavior.
2. An understanding that addiction is a primary, chronic, multi-faceted disease characterized by loss of control of the use of substances in spite of negative consequences.
3. Long-term and short-term treatment goals are specified.
4. The principles of Alcoholics Anonymous and Narcotics Anonymous are fundamental to recovery. (Boise CareUnit, 1997:54)

Client involvement in their own treatment is regarded as a prerequisite for successful rehabilitation/habilitation programming. In the SICI RSAT program inmate-clients are intimately engaged in decisions regarding their own and one another's treatment programming because they are involved in the selection of their own leaders or coordinators, problem solving related to their own high-risk behaviors, and maintenance of community and programmatic integrity through the use of "push-ups," "pull-ups," and even "haircuts" to encourage or discourage behavior by group members (CompCare, 1998).

Aftercare that provides a continuum of care for therapeutic community members is highly regarded by researchers as a means of ensuring a more prosocial transition for offenders (Bowman et al., 1997; Hartmann et al., 1997; McMurran, 1995). The SICI RSAT program is engaged in solidifying the development of an aftercare program that will be structured and provide graduates with a continuum of care. Participant aftercare plans, although integral to successful programming, are not part of these current inmate evaluations of programming.

RSAT Process Evaluation Issues

As indicated by the literature, fashioning a valid evaluation of substance abuse programming is possible but problematic (Anglin & Speckart, 1988; Chen & Rossi, 1980; Field, 1985, 1989; Finney et al., 1981; Fletcher & Tims, 1992; Henning & Frueh, 1996; Inciardi, Martin, Lockwood, Hooper, & Wald, 1992; Incorvaia & Kirby, 1997; Lipton, Pearson, & Wexler, 1997; Pelissier & McCarthy, 1992; Sannibale, 1989; Wexler & Williams, 1986; Wexler, Falkin, Lipton, & Rosenblum, 1992; Wolk & Hartmann, 1996). Program evaluation entails the need to attend to the "process" of the treatment before the outcomes might be truly measured. As Wolk and Hartmann (1996:70) indicate, "The primary goal of a process evaluation is to establish and maintain program integrity."

Establishing and maintaining program integrity requires rigorous examination of a number of program components and provider and participant activity and preparedness over a period of time (Inciardi et al., 1992; Fletcher & Tims, 1992; Lipton et al., 1997; Wolk & Hartmann, 1996). A process evaluation provides the opportunity for providers to become attuned to the basic strengths and weaknesses of the program during and after this initial implementation period. Key to this tuning process is attention to the details of program goals and objectives, admittance and release criteria and procedures, program requirements of inmates, treatment and custody staff training and perspective, program content connection to established and viable treatment protocols, prison administration involvement and support, parole board commitment, and provision for aftercare treatment (Inciardi et al., 1992; Wexler & Williams, 1986; Wolk & Hartmann, 1996).

The methods used to investigate such matters include program visitation and observation; archival research on program manuals, policies, procedures, staff training, inmate assessment, intake and exit instruments; data review from the inmate management system; interviews of key actors; review of aftercare procedures and content; and surveys of staff and inmates on their satisfaction with, and perceptions of, programmatic success. As indicated earlier, we will focus here on inmate survey data.

METHODS

The inmate questionnaire was created by the researchers after a review of the literature and revised after observation of the program operation. The instrument items were analyzed for face validity. Procedures included separate readings of the instrument by the authors and several corrections administrators. Items that did not seem to adequately address an issue were revised per the suggestions of the readers. We were particularly interested in how the inmate participants perceived the content of the various components of the program and the delivery of that content, how the inmate coordinators and staff treatment personnel were viewed, whether the inmates thought the tools of a true therapeutic community were present and operating well, whether communication lines were open and positive, and what was their perception of the quality of services delivered and the likely effect of those services on participants. Reliability is discussed in a later section.

A fifty-one-item Likert scale instrument was created to measure these perceptions of the RSAT program. Inmates were also asked to provide some demographic information, queried regarding their substance use and abuse, and given the opportunity to provide written comments about the strengths and weaknesses of the program.

The questionnaire was distributed to all participants at one meeting in fall 1999. Neither treatment nor security staff were apprised of the content of the questionnaire, nor were they present at the time of the administration. The questionnaire was administered by one of the researchers on the project. Completion of the questionnaire was voluntary and no information that would allow us to identify a particular inmate was solicited. Forty-two of the forty-five inmates present at the meeting chose to fill out the questionnaire. There are forty-eight inmates in the RSAT program, three of which were unable to attend the meeting. Excluding these three inmates, we achieved a response rate of 93.3 percent, or virtually every inmate enrolled in the program.

For the analysis a total of thirteen of the original fifty-one items were reverse coded for ease of interpretation. Thus, for all items, the higher the mean, the more positive the assessment of a given program component.

FINDINGS AND ANALYSIS

The inmate demographics (see Table 6.1) reveal that the RSAT inmates are overwhelmingly white (85.7 percent) and non-Hispanic (88.1 percent). This is reflective of the Idaho population generally. RSAT inmates range in age from twenty to fifty, with a mean age of 30.7. Roughly half (45.2 percent) are between the ages of twenty and

TABLE 6.1. Respondent demographics

Demographic variable	N	%
Race		
White	36	85.7
Black	1	2.4
Multiracial	2	4.8
Other	2	4.8
Ethnicity		
Hispanic	3	7.1
Non-Hispanic	37	88.1
Age*		
20-24	10	23.8
25-29	9	21.4
30-34	12	28.6
35+	11	26.2
Education		
Less than HS diploma	4	9.5
HS diploma	28	66.7
Some college	6	14.3
AA degree	4	9.5
College degree	0	0.0

Note: Some respondents did not answer every question.

*Mean age = 30.69, SD = 7.33; age range: 20-50.

twenty-nine. A significant portion (26.2 percent) are at least thirty-five years old. In accord with national-level data, the RSAT inmate population is relatively undereducated. Approximately three-quarters (76.2 percent) have no more than a high school diploma or GED, and none have a four-year college degree.

The Idaho RSAT program is intended to last nine months and consists of three distinct phases through which the inmate moves. Each phase is designed to last three months. Successful completion of one phase allows the inmate to move to the next phase; failure to successfully complete a phase leads to termination from the program or repetition of that phase. In the present sample, the majority (83.4 percent) of respondents were in either Phase 1 or Phase 2 (see Table 6.2). The amount of time spent in RSAT ranges from one month to nine months, with a roughly equal distribution across the first six months of the program. The mean number of months in the program for all respondents was 4.3.

Advanced RSAT inmates (those in the Phase 3) may become inmate coordinators. Inmate coordinators lead some of the group meetings and act as facilitators and leaders. Perhaps because they were afraid they could be identified by their response to the status question, only twenty-seven inmates identified themselves as a participant or a coordinator.

The RSAT inmates were asked several questions regarding their substance abuse history prior to incarceration. As Table 6.3 indicates, alcohol and drug use are common among the respondents. This comes as no surprise. What is interesting is the amount of drug and alcohol use to which the respondents admitted. Only one inmate claimed to have never used drugs. A majority (59.5 percent) of inmates got high daily, while another 16.7 percent got high at least once per week. Only 16.7 percent of the inmates got drunk on a daily basis, although 38.2 percent consumed alcohol daily. These data suggest that drugs are the substance of choice among this population but that most of these respondents also used alcohol. In fact, these findings indicate that almost 93 percent of the respondents were sometimes or always high when they committed crimes.

We next performed a reliability analysis on the fifty-one Likert scale items. As reported in Table 6.4, the alpha for the entire scale was found to be a robust .9324 (Babbie, 1992). We also performed a reliability analysis on portions of the survey instrument, each of which was intended to measure a particular aspect of the RSAT program. These include perceptions of program content and delivery (thirteen items after two were removed), perceptions of treatment leader and

TABLE 6.2. Respondent RSAT data

Participant progress	N	%
Months in RSAT*		
1	5	11.9
2	7	16.7
3	5	11.9
4	5	11.9
6	7	16.7
7	3	7.1
8	2	4.8
9	2	4.8
RSAT phase		
First	17	40.5
Second	18	42.9
Third	6	14.3
Cognitive Self-Change Program		
CSC 1	17	40.5
CSC 2	19	45.2
CSC 3	6	14.3
RSAT status		
Participant	23	54.8
Coordinator	4	9.5

Note: Some respondents did not answer every question.

*Mean months in RSAT = 4.30, SD = 2.35

involvement issues (eight items after one was removed), perceptions of the therapeutic atmosphere (sixteen items), and perceptions of quality of service (eleven items). The alpha for each of these portions of the questionnaire ranged from .7017 to .8466 (see Table 6.4).

TABLE 6.3. Respondent prior substance abuse

Inmate responses	N	%
Alcohol use		
Never	4	9.5
1 drink per month	8	19.0
1-2 drinks per week	13	31.0
1-2 drinks per day	7	16.7
3-5 drinks per day	2	4.8
Got drunk daily	7	16.7
Total	41	
Drug use		
Never	1	2.4
1 fix per month	9	21.4
1-2 fixes per week	7	16.7
1 fix per day	25	59.5
Total	42	
Relationship between substance abuse and crime		
Never high	3	7.1
Sometimes high	12	28.6
Always high	27	64.3
Total	42	

Note: Some respondents did not answer every question.

Inmates' Perceptions of RSAT Programming

We next examined the data related to the mean and standard deviations for each of the four reference subscales, using one-way analysis of variance (ANOVA) to determine significant differences by age, education, current programming phase, and inmates' self-reported frequency of use of alcohol/drugs prior to incarceration. Those findings are reported in Tables 6.5 through 6.8.

TABLE 6.4. Reliability analysis

Scale	Alpha
Entire 51-item instrument	.9324
Subscale #1 Perceptions of program content and delivery (13 items: 12-26, 17 and 21 out)	.7454
Subscale #2 Perceptions of treatment leader and involvement issues (8 items: 27-35, 31 out)	.7017
Subscale #3 Perceptions of the therapeutic atmosphere (16 items: 36-51)	.8466
Subscale #4 Perceptions of quality of service (11 items: 52-62)	.8405

As indicated in these tables, most of the respondents were quite positive in their assessments of the RSAT program operation. In three of the four categories of items, perceptions of program content and delivery (subscale 1, Table 6.5), perceptions of treatment leader and involvement issues (subscale 2, Table 6.6), and perceptions of quality of service and communication issues (subscale 4, Table 6.8), the overall mean for all respondents was in the top quarter of the range of possible responses. Two of these subscales, numbers 2 and 4, were also within the top fifth of possible mean responses. In general, these findings do indicate that the inmate participants are generally positive regarding the treatment program they are experiencing.

However, on the third subscale, perceptions of the therapeutic atmosphere, and to a lesser degree the first subscale, perceptions of program content and delivery, the inmate participants were slightly less positive in their assessment of the program. Subscale 3 items were directed at trust, assistance, and encouragement issues and whether they felt a sense of a community in the program (Table 6.7). Since the therapeutic community concept is core to this RSAT program, this finding is an important indicator of an area meriting attention by program delivery personnel. To the extent that this lower relative mean on subscale 3 may be related to a lack of trust, it may also be an indicator of the difficulties inherent in the delivery of a true

TABLE 6.5. Subscale #1: Perceptions of program content and delivery

Category	N	Mean	Standard deviation	F	p
Age					
20-24	4	48.3	5.74		
25-29	7	51.1	7.46		
30-34	12	50.7	9.06		
35+	10	52.8	3.33	.431	.732
Education					
HS or less	24	52.1	5.76		
Some college	9	48.6	8.99	1.793	.190
RSAT phase					
Phase 1	13	54.9[a]	3.95		
Phase 2	14	46.5[b]	7.27		
Phase 3	6	53.7	4.23	8.183	.001
Alcohol use					
Rarely or never use	18	51.3	6.47		
Moderate drinker	8	49.6	5.71		
Heavy drinker	7	52.3	9.32	.290	.751
Drug use					
Rarely use	8	52.9[a]	6.66		
Moderate user	6	44.8[b]	8.23		
Heavy user	18	52.4	5.68	3.519	.043

Note: Range 13 to 65, mean for all categories = 50.8, within the top quartile at 48.8 of possible means for responses, but not within the top quintile at 52.

[a]Statistically significant differences between Phase 1 and Phase 2 or between Categories 1 and 2 at the .10 level.

[b]Statistically significant differences between Phase 2 and Phase 3 or between Categories 2 and 3 at the .10 level.

TABLE 6.6. Subscale #2: Perceptions of treatment leader and involvement issues

Category	N	Mean	Standard deviation	F	p
Age					
20-24	9	32.3	3.67		
25-29	9	31.6	5.61		
30-34	12	32.5	5.57		
35+	10	33.6	4.06	.287	.834
Education					
HS or less	30	33.0	4.22		
Some college	10	31.0	5.98	1.404	.243
RSAT phase					
Phase 1	17	34.1	3.75		
Phase 2	17	30.9	5.60		
Phase 3	6	32.7	3.50	1.945	.157
Alcohol use					
Rarely or never use	24	31.5	4.81		
Moderate drinker	7	31.9	5.08		
Heavy drinker	9	35.9*	2.52	3.317	.047
Drug use					
Rarely use	8	35.0	2.56		
Moderate user	7	30.6	6.43		
Heavy user	24	32.3	4.66	1.749	.188

Note: Range 8 to 40, mean for all categories = 32.6, within the top quartile at 30.0 and top quintile at 32 of possible means for responses.

*Statistically significant differences between Categories 1 and 3 at the .10 level.

TABLE 6.7. Subscale #3: Perceptions of the therapeutic atmosphere

Category	N	Mean	Standard deviation	F	p
Age					
20-24	6	55.3	8.89		
25-29	6	54.8	14.08		
30-34	10	57.0	12.02		
35+	8	59.6	8.50	.271	.846
Education					
HS or less	21	57.1	10.00		
Some college	9	56.6	12.70	.016	.901
RSAT phase					
Phase 1	14	59.3	6.87		
Phase 2	11	51.1*	13.5		
Phase 3	5	63.2	6.80	3.317	.052
Alcohol use					
Rarely use	18	55.5	11.50		
Moderate drinker	5	55.2	9.68		
Heavy drinker	7	61.9	8.65	.975	.390
Drug use					
Rarely or never use	5	62.2	10.57		
Moderate user	6	54.2	14.00		
Heavy user	19	56.4	9.65	.825	.449

Note: Range 16 to 80, mean for all categories = 57.3, not within the quartile at 60 or top quintile at 64 of possible means for responses.

*Statistically significant differences between Phase 2 and Phase 3 or between Categories 2 and 3 at the .10 level.

TABLE 6.8. Subscale #4: Perceptions of quality of service and communication issues

Category	N	Mean	Standard deviation	F	p
Age					
20-24	7	44.4	6.40		
25-29	7	44.3	7.57		
30-34	11	44.5	6.22		
35+	7	46.6	4.23	.223	.880
Education					
HS or less	25	45.3	5.71		
Some college	7	43.3	7.16	.624	.436
RSAT phase					
Phase 1	15	47.1*	4.67		
Phase 2	12	42.0	7.03		
Phase 3	5	45.2	4.76	2.650	.088
Alcohol use					
Rarely use	20	43.8	6.49		
Moderate drinker	4	45.0	4.55		
Heavy drinker	8	47.5	4.93	1.099	.347
Drug use					
Rarely or never use	5	46.0	6.63		
Moderate user	4	39.5	7.33		
Heavy user	22	45.5	5.50	1.857	.175

Note: Range 11 to 55, mean for all categories = 44.7, within the top quarter at 41.3 and top quintile at 44 of possible means for responses.

*Statistically significant differences between Phase 1 and Phase 2 or between Categories 1 and 2 at the .10 level.

therapeutic community in a correctional environment. That is, the operation of the therapeutic community requires trust, yet the operation of a prison and the security concerns that prevail with inmate populations necessarily require distrust. Such different perspectives may never be completely reconcilable.

The ANOVA analysis of the four subscales by selected age, education, RSAT phase status, and alcohol and drug use categories is also displayed in Tables 6.5 through 6.8. As the data reveal, neither age nor education had a significant effect on inmate perceptions on any of the four subscales. The only variables that did have statistically significant relationship was the RSAT phases on subscales 3 and 4, alcohol use categories on subscale 2, and drug use categories on subscale 1.

Inmates in the third RSAT phase had a higher mean score than those in the second or first phase on subscale 3, while inmates in the first RSAT phase had a higher mean score than those in the second or third phase on subscale 4. In both cases, the first and third phase people were more positive in their perceptions of the program than were the people in the middle or second phase of the program. Closer examination of inmates in the program indicates that those in the second phase score consistently lower than those in either Phase 1 or Phase 3. The result is a U-shaped curve, similar to the U-shaped curve often found in studies on prisonization and inmate socialization (Berk, 1968; Garabedian, 1963; Wellford, 1967; Wheeler, 1961). Wheeler (1961) measured the attitudes of inmates who had spent varying degrees of time in prison, to determine if the degree of prisonization differed based on the amount of time served. He found that inmate attitudes tended to conform to staff norms and expectations at both the beginning and near the end of their sentence. He felt that the U-shaped curve could be explained by the inmate's response to prison—at first the inmate internalizes the societal rejection implicit in his status as a convict, resulting in lower self-esteem. After a period of time, the inmate adjusts his picture of himself and begins to reject social conformity and adopt support for the inmate subculture, which rejects conventional values. This allows the inmate to restore his self-esteem.

The findings on drug and alcohol use categories—the heavy and rare drug users were more positive in their perceptions than were the moderate users on subscale 1, and the heavy alcohol users were more positive in their perceptions than were the rare drinkers on subscale 2—is an encouraging sign for the program. It indicates that those who need treatment the most, those who are heavy substance abusers (those who drink three to five drinks per day or get drunk daily and/or those who got a fix every day) were also those who tended to perceive the program more positively on these subscales.

Predicting Inmates' Attitudes Toward RSAT Programming

We next conducted a series of regression analyses to measure the extent to which the amount of variance in inmates' perceptions of RSAT programming can be explained by months in treatment and self-reported frequency of use of drugs and alcohol. We entered the variables alcohol use, drug use, and months in RSAT (as a proxy for phases) into five regression equations: the entire fifty-one-item scale, and the four subscales. We performed a stepwise backward elimination on each equation. As shown in Table 6.9, and with only one exception, nothing remained in any equation. The exception was Model 3 (subscale 2). In this model, alcohol use (standardized beta of .285) and months in the program (standardized beta of −.346) remained in the equation, with an adjusted R square of .161.

These findings indicate that those in the program longest have a negative view of this particular portion of it, the treatment and leader and involvement issues subscale. Conversely, those with the most serious pattern of alcohol abuse are more likely to view these subscale items in a positive light. Notably, the effect of these two variables, negative for months in the program and positive for alcohol abuse, are fairly constant for all the models (with the exception of months on Model 4), albeit not statistically significant. As this particular subscale includes items concerned with the preparation of treatment leaders, the participation of inmates and staff, and the assistance and encouragement that inmates provide to one another, closer examination of the particular atmosphere of the treatment environment is merited. The finding on alcohol is actually a positive one for the program, again indicating that those who perhaps need the program most are also those who value this portion of it most. However, we would note that the number of inmates who indicated they were what we would characterize as heavy drinkers included only nine inmates out of the forty-two respondents.

TABLE 6.9. Regression on the entire instrument and the four subscales

Model	Unstandardized coefficients B	Standard error	Standardized coefficients beta	t	Adjusted R square	Significance
Model 1[a]						
Constant	175.736	39.129		4.491		.001
Months	-1.514	2.784	-.139	-.544		.595
Alcohol	4.504	4.239	.284	1.062		.306
Drugs	2.451	8.790	.075	.279	.000	.784
Model 2[b]						
Constant	58.862	6.728		8.005		.000
Months	-.712	.526	-.252	-1.353		.187
Alcohol	3.122E-02	.866	.007	.036		.972
Drugs	-3.475E-02	1.436	-.005	-.024	.000	.981
Model 3[c]						
Constant	32.359	2.140		15.121		.000
Months	-.670	.292	-.346	-2.296		.028

Alcohol	.851	.450	.285	1.892	.161	.067

Model 4[d]						
Constant	58.597	12.331		4.752		.000
Months	.335	.869	.077	.385		.703
Alcohol	.843	1.370	.126	.615		.544
Drugs	-1.726	2.890	-.125	-.597	.000	.556
Model 5[e]						
Constant	41.008	6.729		6.094		.000
Months	-.126	.479	-.051	-.264		.794
Alcohol	.869	.765	.229	1.135		.267
Drugs	.337	1.368	.049	.246	.000	.807

[a]All perceptions model (items 12 to 62, by alcohol use, drug use, months in program).
[b]First subscale (items 12 to 26, by alcohol use, drug use, months in program).
[c]Second subscale (items 27 to 35, by alcohol use, drug use, months in program).
[d]Third subscale (items 36 to 51, by alcohol use, drug use, months in program).
[e]Fourth subscale (items 52 to 62, by alcohol use, drug use, months in program).

Identified Strengths and Weaknesses of RSAT Programming by the Inmates

In addition to answering the Likert scale items, the RSAT inmates were asked to identify the strengths and weaknesses of the RSAT program. Responses to these two items revealed a variety of complaints and positive comments. A content analysis of the responses revealed that the most commonly listed strengths included the Narcotics Anonymous and Alcoholics Anonymous meetings (fifteen responses), the counselors (eleven responses), the feelings of fellowship among the community members (nine responses), the support system (eight responses), and the therapeutic community atmosphere (eight responses).

The most commonly listed weaknesses included the presence of people who retaliated against others (eight responses), the prison location of the TC (five responses), petty requirements and rules (five responses), and poor CSC (cognitive self-change) instructors (five responses). Obviously, some of the strengths listed by some inmate participants are listed as weaknesses by other inmates. This ambivalence was somewhat reflected in the ANOVA and regression analysis. In general, the respondents were positive in their assessment of the program in total, but that support varied by program component (the subscales), by status in the program (phases and months in), and by individual characteristics of the inmates (alcohol use and drug use).

The findings reported here indicate that the inmate participants in this RSAT program generally perceive it in a positive light. Moreover, those with the most serious pattern of alcohol abuse are more positive about it. Why this is not true for the more numerous drug offenders is not clear. However, these findings are tempered by the knowledge that those in the program longest are generally less positive about it relative to those just entering the program. We suspect this finding is in part tied to the continuous-enrollment policy of this program. This policy is in place to ensure that the program is always full or nearly full. Because of this policy, those in one of the first two phases are re-exposed to some of the same information again and again as new participants are admitted to that phase. By the third phase, many of the inmate participants may be more positive about the program as they are afforded the opportunity to work as inmate coordinators and are given more freedom to work off-site. This phenomena is only complemented by the U-shaped prisonization effect common in prison environs.

CONCLUSIONS AND POLICY RECOMMENDATIONS

Our general conclusion is that this RSAT program is framed and operated in a manner that befits its organizational and programmatic mandates to deliver substance abuse and cognitive self-change programming in a therapeutic community environment. Program content included in-depth programming on cognitive self-change, twelve-step programming, and the traditions, boundaries, and reinforcement of behaviors that typify a therapeutic community. Attributes of this program that reflected successful programming in the literature included cognitive processes and practice (e.g., journaling or thinking reports, CSC groups, and process groups), prosocial modeling by staff and inmate coordinators, intensive engagement in their own treatment by clients, the presence of a therapeutic community environment, and external support from the prison staff and administration, the corrections department, and the parole authority. It is the research team's belief that this program is likely to result in less recidivism and reduced costs for taxpayers.

Our data indicate that if the staff are trained and experienced, the facilities are adequate, the program is operated as a true therapeutic community, and the cognitive self-change component is developed and practiced, an RSAT program will be perceived positively by inmate participants. Of course, the perceptions of the staff who deliver these programs, particularly when private-sector entities pay less and provide fewer benefits and opportunities for training, are another matter that merits study, but we did not measure that here.

As a means of improving an existing program, we offer the following recommendations, based on our observation of this RSAT program.

1. Extensive cognitive self-change and therapeutic community training be provided to both the treatment providers and the correctional staff
2. Correctional staff be provided with educational programming that will enhance their understanding of the RSAT program and its TC environment
3. The pay for treatment personnel be commensurate with their qualifications and skills
4. Additional programming that addresses the collateral needs of inmate clients be offered, such as anger management, relationship management, parenting, and dealing with sexual abuse

5. Including "trust building" exercises between and among the inmate-clients as a means of reinforcing the community
6. Opportunities (e.g., meetings, training sessions, or even social events) be created that will enhance the positive communication and interactions between counselors and correctional officers
7. The TC environment be strengthened with structural and environmental changes, such as placing the program in more isolated quarters, employing the use of softer furnishings and less institutional paint and accoutrements, establishing a resource library, and allowing gathering in a common area on an informal basis. We believe, based on the literature on TCs and that on other innovative correctional environments, such as podular/direct-supervision jails, that such changes will convey the clear message that this is a community- and treatment-oriented environment, as well as a correctional one.
8. Aftercare be provided for inmates. RSAT alone is clearly not enough. Continued treatment and services in the community are required.

For corrections administrators considering the implementation of an RSAT program, we strongly urge an extensive review of existing programs, such as the one under study here, so that they may learn from those who have gone before. In addition to the suggestions we have made, we would urge administrators considering new RSAT programs to ensure that the infrastructure is in place before the program begins. This means, at the very least, finding funding for additional treatment staff, space for the TC, adequate educational and programmatic materials, and resources for aftercare.

Within the institution, administrators must work to obtain, train, and keep qualified treatment staff. In addition, security staff must be brought online. If security staff are not educated about the program and convinced to buy in to the TC, their resistance will greatly impact on the ability of the TC to thrive. While training the treatment staff is obviously important, educating the security staff is an oft-overlooked, but vital, task.

Administrators must also do what they can to solicit inmate feedback on the program. A true TC requires communication among all the parties. Inmate feedback should be sought on not only the content of the program but also the delivery. As our research indicates, program delivery can vary greatly from one day to the next and from one person to the next. It is crucial that administrators are aware of inmate perceptions of the TC, for if inmates do not believe in it, it is doomed to failure.

Finally, it must be said that administrators need to be open to suggestions and criticism from persons they are not used to listening closely to. All the stakeholders, including inmates, must have a voice. After all, one of the tenets of a therapeutic community and of successful treatment programming is inmate involvement in their own habilitation. If we are to reinforce such practices, and if we are to get a true picture of program operation, we should ask those who know it best and experience it most, and that would be the inmate participants.

DISCUSSION QUESTIONS

1. Why do Stohr and associates view the Residential Substance Abuse Treatment (RSAT) Programming described here as different from the type of programming that is described in the Arkansas therapeutic community by both Golden (Chapter 4) and Patenaude (Chapter 5)?
2. Why, according to these authors, do correctional programs sometimes fail to meet their goals?
3. What explanation do Stohr and associates give for their finding that inmates who are in the RSAT program longer hold more negative feelings about the program overall than do inmates just entering the program?
4. These authors offer some concrete recommendations for substance abuse treatment programming in the institutional environment. How would you summarize those recommendations?

APPENDIX: IDAHO RSAT CLIENT QUESTIONNAIRE

In this questionnaire we ask key program stakeholders, such as yourself, questions that will provide the RSAT process evaluators with a general sense about how the RSAT program at SICI is operating. Although participation in answering these questions is completely voluntary and anonymous (we do not need your name on this survey), we would ask you to kindly respond to these questions so that the RSAT program might be delivered in the most effective manner.

Demographics

1. Status (please circle the correct answer): Coordinator/Participant
2. Number of months in SICI RSAT program: _____
3. Which cognitive self-change program are you currently in? (put an X in front of the correct answer)
   _____ CSC 1
   _____ CSC 2
   _____ CSC 3
   _____ Other (please explain)_____
4. Which phase of the RSAT program are you currently in? (please write in the correct phase)
   Phase _____
5. Race (please circle the answer that best describes you):
   a.   White
   b.   Black (African American)
   c.   Asian
   d.   American Indian
   e.   Multiracial
   f.   Other _____
6. Ethnicity (please circle the answer that best describes you):
   a.   Hispanic
   b.   Non-Hispanic
7. Age: _____
8. Amount of education (please circle the answer that best describes you):
   a.   8 years or less
   b.   Less than high school or GED
   c.   High school or GED
   d.   Some college or technical degree
   e.   Associate's degree
   f.   Bachelor's degree
   g.   Master's degree or more
9. Use of alcohol prior to incarceration (please circle the answer that best describes you):
   a.   I never used alcohol before incarcerated this last time.
   b.   I had about a drink once per month before incarcerated this last time.
   c.   I had a drink or two per week before incarcerated this last time.

    d.   I had a drink or two per day before incarcerated this last time.

    e.   I had three to five drinks per day before incarcerated this last time.

    f.   I would drink to get drunk daily, or as often as I could, before incarcerated this last time.

10. Use of illegal drugs prior to incarceration (please circle the answer that best describes you):

    a.   I never used illegal drugs before incarcerated this last time.

    b.   I had about one fix per month of illegal drugs before incarcerated this last time.

    c.   I had one fix or two per week of illegal drugs before incarcerated this last time.

    d.   I got a fix every day, or as often as I could, of illegal drugs before incarcerated this last time.

11. Relationship between substance abuse (alcohol or illegal drugs) and criminal behavior (please circle the answer that best describes you):

    a.   I was always high or drunk when I committed a crime.

    b.   I was sometimes high or drunk when I committed a crime.

    c.   I was never high or drunk when I committed a crime.

Perceptions of Program Content and Delivery

On a scale of 1 to 5 please indicate your perception of the truth of the following statements.

1	2	3	4	5
Not true	Somewhat true	Very true	Not applicable	Don't know

12. It is usually easy to understand what the staff treatment personnel are trying to say in groups. _____

13. Presentations by staff treatment personnel are usually well organized with a clear beginning, middle, and end. _____

14. The content of a program rarely reflects the announced subject matter. _____

15. Inmate coordinators are fully prepared to lead the a.m. and p.m. discussions. _____

16. The group meetings rarely end on time. _____

17. Lifting weights and other physical activity helps me to stay focused on changing my life for the better. _____

18. Cognitive self-change groups are useful in that they help me to reflect upon my behavior and thought processes. _____

19. The morning meetings force me to focus on my attitude and my treatment program. _____

20. There is sometimes not enough handbook material to help us prepare for groups. _____

21. The morning meetings' creative energy and learning experience exercises are useful in building a sense of community in the program. _____

22. The AA/NA meetings are usually not that helpful in my treatment. _____

23. When I give a pull-up to another community member, I am really showing responsible concern for that person. _____

24. The p.m. closure meetings help me to put together all the information I learned in that day. _____

25. People who commit criminal acts while abusing alcohol and drugs rarely make errors in criminal thinking. _____

26. My treatment program has pointed out the barriers I put up to avoid changing in a positive way. _____

Perceptions of Treatment Leader and Involvement Issues

On a scale of 1 to 5 please indicate your perception of the truth of the following statements.

27. The treatment staff personnel are usually prepared to lead groups. _____

28. The inmate coordinators are usually prepared to lead the a.m. and p.m. groups. _____

29. Inmates are usually encouraged to participate by the staff treatment personnel or by inmate coordinators. _____

30. Other RSAT inmates sometimes discourage me from sticking with my treatment program. _____

31. Non-RSAT inmates sometimes discourage me from sticking with my treatment program. _____

32. The staff treatment personnel or inmate coordinator usually keeps the program moving along. _____

33. The staff treatment personnel are usually not involved much in program delivery. _____

34. The inmates are usually very involved in program delivery. _____

35. Inmate coordinators usually reinforce prosocial or anticriminal behavior, even in the living unit. _____

Perceptions of the Therapeutic Atmosphere

On a scale of 1 to 5 please indicate your perception of the truth of the following statements.

36. There is usually a sense of trust between correctional staff and inmates in this program. _____
37. Inmates are afraid to complain to correctional staff about treatment issues for fear that they will not be allowed to remain in the program. _____
38. Inmates are afraid to complain to treatment staff about treatment issues for fear that they will not be allowed to remain in the program. _____
39. Pull-ups are given only when the behavior of a TC member requires it. _____
40. Haircuts are given only when a TC member is in danger of failing in the program. _____
41. Encounters are scheduled with an inmate only when his negative behaviors need to be addressed by other community members. _____
42. If I have a problem with sticking to my treatment program there are correctional staff here I can go to for help. _____
43. If I have a problem with sticking to my program there are treatment staff here I can go to for help. _____
44. There is usually a sense of trust between staff treatment personnel and inmates in this program. _____
45. I have an inmate mentor in the program who helps me stick to my treatment plan. _____
46. Treatment staff here freely give push-ups. _____
47. Generally inmates are not sincere in their participation in this program. _____
48. When inmates complain about legitimate treatment issues, their comments are usually ignored. _____
49. Correctional staff here freely give push-ups. _____
50. The pull-ups I've received from this program have taught me how to change in a positive and noncriminal way. _____
51. This RSAT program makes me feel like I am part of a close-knit and supportive community. _____

Quality of Services

On a scale of 1 to 5 please indicate your perception of the truth of the following statements regarding the knowledge and skills that inmates gain from participation in this RSAT program.

1	2	3	4	5
Low	Neutral	High	Not applicable	Don't know

52. How would you rate the level of positive communication between treatment staff and inmates in this program? _____
53. How would you rate the level of positive communication between inmate participants in this program? _____
54. How would you rate the level of consistency in delivery of treatment services by staff treatment personnel? _____
55. How would you rate the level of consistency in delivery of security services by correctional personnel? _____
56. How would you rate the level of physical safety you feel in this program? _____

On a scale of 1 to 5 please indicate your perception of the truth of the following statements.

1	2	3	4	5
Not true	Somewhat true	Very true	Not applicable	Don't know

57. Generally speaking, inmate graduates are more knowledgeable about drug and alcohol abuse after completing this program. _____
58. Inmates *do not* possess more skills or abilities to help them avoid substance abuse after having completed this program. _____
59. Inmates who complete this program are more likely to avoid criminal thinking errors once back in the community. _____
60. Even inmates who complete a portion of this RSAT program are likely to be more successful when on parole than are people with substance abuse problems who didn't participate in this program. _____
61. Even inmates who complete a portion of this RSAT program are more likely to avoid alcohol or drug abuse in the future than are people with substance abuse problems who didn't participate in this program. _____
62. Because of the focus on cognitive self-change programming here, I will be less likely to commit crime while on parole than will those who didn't graduate from this RSAT program. _____

RSAT Strengths and Weaknesses

63. Please identify three strengths of the RSAT treatment program.
    a. _____
    b. _____
    c. _____
64. Please identify three weaknesses of the RSAT treatment program.
    a. _____
    b. _____
    c. _____

REFERENCES

Andrews, D.A., Zinger, I., Hoge, R.D., Bonta, J., Gendreau, P., & Cullen, F.T. (1990). Does correctional treatment work? A clinically relevant and psychologically informed meta-analysis. *Criminology, 28,* 369-404.

Anglin, M.D. & Speckart, G. (1988). Narcotics use and crime: A multisample, multimethod analysis. *Criminology, 26,* 197-233.

Antonowicz, D.H. & Ross, R.R. (1997). Essential components of successful rehabilitation programs for offenders. In J.W. Marquart & J.R. Sorensen (Eds.), *Correctional contexts: Contemporary and classical readings* (pp. 222-247). Los Angeles, CA: Roxbury.

Associated Press. (1998, March 23). Almost half of probationers say drugs, alcohol used before crimes. *Idaho Statesman,* p. A1.

Babbie, E. (1992). *The practice of social research* (6th ed.). Belmont, CA: Wadsworth.

Berk, B.B. (1968). Organizational goals and inmate organization. *American Journal of Sociology, 71,* 522-534.

Boise CareUnit. (1997). *Proposal to provide residential substance abuse treatment (RSAT) program at the South Idaho Correctional Institution.* Boise, ID: Comprehensive Care Integration.

Bowman, V.E., Lowrey, L., & Purser, J. (1997). Two-tiered humanistic pre-release interventions for prison inmates. *Journal of Offender Rehabilitation, 25,* 115-128.

Calco-Gray, E. (1993). The dos pasos: Alternatives to incarceration for substance abusing women of childbearing age. *American Jails, 7,* 44-53.

Cardenas, E.D. (1996). *An evaluation of the implementation, administration and impact of the "Residential Substance Abuse Treatment for State Prisoners Program" at South Idaho Correctional Institution.* Boise: Idaho Department of Correction.

Chen, H. & Rossi, P.H. (1980). The multi-goal, theory-driven approach to evaluation: A model linking basic and applied social science. *Social Forces, 59,* 106-122.

CompCare. (1998). *RSAT inmate handbook*. Boise: Idaho State Correctional Institution.

Corrections Alert. (1998). Therapeutic communities show promise for reducing drug addiction among prisoners. *Corrections Alert, 4,* 1-2.

Cullen, E., Jones, L., & Woodward, R. (Eds.) (1997). *Therapeutic communities for offenders*. New York: John Wiley and Sons.

Early, K.E. (Ed.) (1996). *Drug treatment behind bars: Prison-based strategies for change*. Westport, CT: Praeger.

Farabee, D., Prendergast, M., & Anglin, M.D. (1998). The effectiveness of coerced treatment for drug-abusing offenders. *Federal Probation, 62,* 3-10.

Farabee, D., Prendergast, M., Cartier, J., Wexler, H., Knight, K., & Anglin, M.D. (1999). Barriers to implementing effective correctional drug treatment programs. *The Prison Journal, 79,* 150-162.

Field, G. (1985). The cornerstone program: A client outcome study. *Federal Probation, 49,* 50-55.

Field, G. (1989). The effects of intensive treatment on reducing the criminal recidivism of addicted offenders. *Federal Probation, 53,* 51-56.

Field, G. (1992). Oregon prison drug treatment programs. In C.G. Leukefeld & F.M. Tims (Eds.), *National Institute on Drug Abuse research monograph series: Drug abuse treatment in prisons and jails* (pp. 187-214). Rockville, MD: National Institute on Drug Abuse.

Finney, J.W., Moos, R.H., & Chan, D.H. (1981). Length of stay and program component effects in the treatment of alcoholism: A comparison of two techniques for process analyses. *Journal of Consulting and Clinical Psychology, 49,* 120-131.

Fletcher, B.W. & Tims, F.M. (1992). Methodological issues: Drug abuse treatment in prisons and jails. In C.G. Leukefeld & F.M. Tims (Eds.), *National Institute on Drug Abuse research monograph series: Drug abuse treatment in prisons and jails* (pp. 94-121). Rockville, MD: National Institute on Drug Abuse.

Garabedian, P. (1963). Social roles and processes of socialization in the prison community. *Social Problems 12*(2), 139-152.

Gendreau, P. (1993, November). The principles of effective intervention with offenders. Paper presented at the International Association of Residential and Community Alternatives Conference, Philadelphia, Pennsylvania.

Gendreau, P. & Ross, R.R. (1987). Revivification of rehabilitation: Evidence for the 1980s. *Justice Quarterly, 4,* 349-407.

Gendreau, P. & Ross, R.R. (1995). Correctional treatment: Some recommendations for effective intervention. In K.C. Haas & G.P. Alpert (Eds.), *The dilemmas of corrections: Contemporary readings* (3rd ed.) (pp. 367-380). Prospect Heights, IL: Waveland.

Hanlon, T.E., Nurco, D.N., Bateman, R.W., & O'Grady, K.E. (1999). The relative effects of three approaches to the parole supervision of narcotic addicts and cocaine abusers. *The Prison Journal, 79,* 163-181.

Hartmann, D.J., Wolk, J.L., Johnston, J.S., & Colyer, C.J. (1997). Recidivism and substance abuse outcomes in a prison-based therapeutic community. *Federal Probation, 51,* 18-25.

Henning, K.R. & Frueh, B.C. (1996). Cognitive-behavioral treatment of incarcerated offenders: An evaluation of the Vermont Department of Corrections' cognitive self-change program. *Criminal Justice and Behavior, 23,* 523-541.

Hiller, M.L., Knight, K., Broome, K.M., & Simpson, D.D. (1998). Legal pressure and treatment retention in a national sample of long-term residential programs. *Criminal Justice and Behavior, 25,* 463-481.

Husband, S.D. & Platt, J.J. (1993). The cognitive skills component in substance abuse treatment in correctional settings: A brief review. *The Journal of Drug Issues, 23,* 31-42.

Inciardi, J.A. (1995). The therapeutic community: An effective model for corrections-based drug abuse treatment. In K.C. Haas & G.P. Alpert (Eds.), *The dilemmas of corrections: Contemporary readings* (3rd ed.) (pp. 406-417). Prospect Heights, IL: Waveland.

Inciardi, J.A., Martin S.S., Lockwood, D., Hooper, R.M., & Wald, B.M. (1992). Obstacles to the implementation and evaluation of drug treatment programs in correctional settings: Reviewing the Delaware key experience. In C.G. Leukefeld & F.M. Tims (Eds.), *National Institute on Drug Abuse research monograph series: Drug abuse treatment in prisons and jails* (pp. 270-291). Rockville, MD: National Institute on Drug Abuse.

Incorvaia, D. & Kirby, N. (1997). A formative evaluation of a drug-free unit in a correctional setting. *International Journal of Offender Therapy and Comparative Criminology, 41,* 231-249.

Knight, K., Simpson, D.D., Chatham, L.R., & Camacho, L.M. (1997). An assessment of prison-based drug treatment: Texas' in-prison therapeutic community program. *Journal of Offender Rehabilitation, 24,* 75-100.

Knight, K., Simpson, D.D., & Hiller, M.L. (1999). Three-year reincarceration outcomes for in-prison therapeutic community treatment in Texas. *The Prison Journal, 79,* 337-351.

Lemieux, C.M. (1998). Determinants of expectation of treatment efficacy among incarcerated substance abusers. *International Journal of Offender Therapy and Comparative Criminology, 42,* 233-245.

Leukefeld, C.G. & Tims, F.M. (Eds.) (1992). *National Institute on Drug Abuse research monograph series: Drug abuse treatment in prisons and jails.* Rockville, MD: National Institute on Drug Abuse.

Lipton, D. (1998). Treatment for drug abusing offenders during correctional supervision: A nationwide overview. *Journal of Offender Rehabilitation, 26,* 1-46.

Lipton, D., Falkin, G.P., & Wexler, H.K. (1992). Correctional drug abuse treatment in the United States: An overview. In C.G. Leukefeld & F.M. Tims (Eds.), *National Institute on Drug Abuse research monograph series: Drug abuse treatment in prisons and jails* (pp. 3-17). Rockville, MD: National Institute on Drug Abuse.

Lipton, D., Martinson, R., & Wilks, J. (1975). *The effectiveness of correctional treatment: A survey of treatment evaluation studies.* Springfield, MA: Praeger.

Lipton, D.S., Pearson, F.S., & Wexler, H.K. (1997). Standards of evaluability. Unpublished document. New York: National Development and Research Institutes.

Lockwood, D., McCorkel, J., & Inciardi, J.A. (1998). Developing comprehensive prison-based therapeutic community treatment for women. *Drugs and Society, 13,* 193-212.

Logan, C.H. & Gaes, G.G. (1993). Meta-analysis and the rehabilitation of punishment. *Justice Quarterly, 10,* 245-263.

Martin, S.S., Butzin, C.A., Saum, C.A., & Inciardi, J.A. (1999). Three-year outcomes of therapeutic community treatment for drug-involved offenders in Delaware: From prison to work release to aftercare. *The Prison Journal, 79,* 294-320.

Martinson, R. (1974). What works? Questions and answers about prison reform. *Public Interest, 35,* 22-54.

McCorkel, J., Harrison, L.D., & Inciardi, J.A. (1998). How treatment is constructed among graduates and dropouts in a prison therapeutic community for women. *Journal of Offender Rehabilitation, 27,* 37-59.

McMurran, M. (1995). Alcohol interventions in prisons: Towards guiding principles for effective intervention. *Psychology, Crime & Law, 1,* 215-226.

McMurran, M., Egan, V., & Ahmadi, S. (1998). A retrospective evaluation of a therapeutic community for mentally disordered offenders. *The Journal of Forensic Psychiatry, 9,* 103-113.

National Center on Addiction and Substance Abuse at Columbia University. (1998). CASA study shows alcohol and drugs implicated in the crimes and incarceration of 80% of men and women in prison. Available at <http://www.casacolumbia.org/media/press/010898.htm>.

National Institute of Corrections. (1997). *Effective interventions with high risk offenders: A NIC Interdivisional What Works Committee seminar.* Longmont, CO: National Institute of Corrections.

Office of Justice Programs. (1998). *Residential substance abuse treatment for state prisoners.* Washington, DC: U.S. Department of Justice.

Palmer, T. (1995). The effectiveness issue today: An overview. In K.C. Haas & G.P. Alpert (Eds.), *The dilemmas of corrections: Contemporary readings* (3rd ed.) (pp. 351-366). Prospect Heights, IL: Waveland.

Pearson, F.S. & Lipton, D.S. (1999). A meta-analytic review of the effectiveness of corrections-based treatments for drug abuse. *The Prison Journal, 79,* 384-410.

Pelissier, B. & McCarthy, D. (1992). Evaluation of the Federal Bureau of Prisons' drug treatment programs. In C.G. Leukefeld & F.M. Tims (Eds.), *National Institute on Drug Abuse research monograph series: Drug abuse treatment in prisons and jails* (pp. 33-49). Rockville, MD: National Institute on Drug Abuse.

Pollock, J. (1997). Rehabilitation revisited. In J. Pollock (Ed.), *Prisons: Today and tomorrow* (pp. 158-216). Gaithersburg, MD: Aspen.

Rice, J.S. & Remy, L.L. (1998). Impact of horticultural therapy on psychosocial functioning among urban jail inmates. *Journal of Offender Rehabilitation, 26,* 169-191.

Rouse, J.J. (1991). Evaluation research on prison-based drug treatment programs and some policy implications. *International Journal of the Addictions, 26,* 29-44.

Sannibale, C. (1989). A prospective study of treatment outcome with a group of male problem drinkers. *Journal of Studies on Alcohol, 50,* 236-244.

Schuiteman, J.G. & Bogle, T.G. (1996). *Evaluation of the Department of Corrections' Indian Creek Therapeutic Community: Progress report*. Richmond, VA: The Criminal Justice Research Center, Virginia Department of Criminal Justice Services.

Siegal, H.A., Wang, J., Carlson, R.G., Falck, R.S., Rahman, A.M., & Fine, R.L. (1999). Ohio's prison-based therapeutic community treatment programs for substance abusers: Preliminary analysis of re-arrest data. *Journal of Offender Rehabilitation, 28*, 33-48.

Smith, J. & Faubert, M. (1990). Programming and process in prisoner rehabilitation: A prison mental health center. *Journal of Offender Counseling, Services and Rehabilitation, 15*, 131-153.

State of Idaho. (1998). *Residential substance abuse treatment for state prisoners application*. Boise, ID: Department of Law Enforcement.

Tims, F.M. & Leukefeld, C.G. (1992). The challenge of drug abuse treatment in prisons and jails. In C.G. Leukefeld & F.M. Tims (Eds.), *National Institute on Drug Abuse research monograph series: Drug abuse treatment in prisons and jails* (pp. 18-32). Rockville, MD: National Institute on Drug Abuse.

Wellford, C. (1967). Factors associated with adoption of the inmate code: A study of normative socialization. *The Journal of Criminal Law, Criminology and Police Science, 58*, 197-203.

Wexler, H.K. (1995). The success of therapeutic communities for substance abusers in American prisons. *Journal of Psychoactive Drugs, 27*, 57-66.

Wexler, H.K., DeLeon, G., Thomas, G., Kressel, D., & Peters, J. (1999). The Amity Prison TC evaluation: Reincarceration outcomes. *Criminal Justice and Behavior, 26*, 147-167.

Wexler, H.K., Falkin, G.P., Lipton, D.S., & Rosenblum, A.B. (1992). Outcome evaluation of a prison therapeutic community for substance abuse treatment. In C.G. Leukefeld & F.M. Tims (Eds.), *National Institute on Drug Abuse research monograph series: Drug abuse treatment in prisons and jails* (pp. 248-262). Rockville, MD: National Institute on Drug Abuse.

Wexler, H.K., Melnick, G., Lowe, L., & Peters, J. (1999). Three-year reincarceration outcomes for Amity in-prison therapeutic community and aftercare in California. *The Prison Journal, 79*, 321-336.

Wexler, H.K. & Williams, R. (1986). The Stay 'n Out therapeutic community: Prison treatment for substance abusers. *Journal of Psychoactive Drugs, 18*, 221-230.

Wheeler, S. (1961). Socialization in correctional communities. *American Sociological Review, 26*, 697-712.

Wolk, J.L. & Hartmann, D.J. (1996). Process evaluation in corrections-based substance abuse treatment. *Journal of Offender Rehabilitation, 23*, 67-78.

Wright, R.A. (1995). Rehabilitation affirmed, rejected, and reaffirmed: Assessments of the effectiveness of offender treatment programs in criminology textbooks, 1956 to 1965 and 1983 to 1992. *Journal of Criminal Justice Education, 6*, 21-41.

PART III:
COMMUNITY-BASED
TREATMENT PROGRAMS

There has been a recognition in the field of corrections of a need for a series of sanctions that fall somewhere between probation and prison. This is because for some prison is too severe a punishment, but regular probation is not severe enough. A continuum of sanctions exists that are community based, including such measures as deemed necessary by corrections managers and supervisors in order to more closely watch those clients who are found to be at a higher risk for re-offending (house arrest, electronic monitoring, and intensive supervision, to name a few). Along with the development of community-based corrections to assist managers in relieving the overcrowding in local and state prisons and jails came the development of community-based treatment programs grounded in the overall goal of reducing reoffending. Just as treatment continues to be one of the many elements of a prison sentence, so too it is now seen as a critical component of the probation and/or parole experience. The following chapters describe programming designed specifically for substance-abusing community corrections clients.

In Chapter 7, Cunningham and Stone introduce data from a local drug court, whose goal it is to reduce recidivism among nonviolent felony offenders who have been arrested for drug possession and who have been found to be addicted to drugs. Chapter 8 by Robert Walker and TK Logan illustrates the "nuts and bolts" of running a drug court, including such critical issues as informed consent, confidentiality, and generally the often strained relationship between the counselor and the client given the requirement of reporting progress and current substance use to the drug court. Sims and DuPont-Morales (Chapter 9) next describe Pennsylvania's Restrictive Intermediate Punishment treatment program that is being used for nonviolent, drug-addicted clients who are being diverted from prison and placed into community substance abuse treatment programs.

Chapter 7

Effects of a Drug Diversion Court on Client Recidivism

Debbie S. Cunningham
William E. Stone

The criminal justice system is continually being challenged in its response to drug crime. Drug law violations still remain the largest percent of all arrests in the United States. According to the U.S. Department of Justice (1995), more than half of all individuals brought into the criminal justice system have substance abuse problems. Although national crime rates in general continue to decline, more than 1.5 million Americans were arrested for drug law violations in 1997, an all-time high. According to the FBI (2000), there was a 36.5 percent increase in arrests for drug abuse violations from 1990 to 1999. However, the criminal justice system has not responded comparatively with an investment in additional jails and courts (Turque, 1989).

In response to this problem, many jurisdictions have begun utilizing drug courts in an effort to reduce the strain on regular criminal courts and to address the underlying problems of addiction. The alternative solution sought with the implementation of drug courts offers nonviolent substance-abusing offenders an effective solution to drugs and drug-related crime. The main purpose of drug courts is to use the authority of the court to reduce crime by changing defendants' drug-using behavior. In exchange for the possibility of dismissed charges or reduced sentences, defendants are diverted to drug court programs. According to the U.S. Department of Justice (1995), two main types of drug courts have evolved: (1) those that expedite the processing of drug cases and (2) those that use court-monitored drug treatment to achieve changes in defendants' drug use. The most prevalent type of drug court is the latter, which combines treatment with adjudication of cases.

DRUG COURT OPERATIONS

The central element of all drug court programs is attendance at the regularly scheduled status hearings at which the drug court judge monitors the progress of participants. Monitoring is based on treatment provider reports, urine test results, attendance at counseling, etc. The judge reinforces progress and addresses noncompliance with program requirements. The primary objective of the status hearing is to keep the defendant in treatment.

Like many of the other characteristics of drug courts, treatment generally varies from jurisdiction to jurisdiction. The treatment services are generally divided into three phases: detoxification, stabilization, and aftercare. According to information supplied by the Drug Court Resource Center to the Committee on the Judiciary (U.S. Department of Justice, 1995), in most drug courts, treatment is designed to usually last at least one year and is administered on an outpatient basis with limited inpatient care as needed to address special detoxification or relapse situations. Sanctions for failing to abide by program rules can include verbal admonition from the judge; demotion to an earlier stage of the program; incarceration for several days or weeks, increasing with the number and severity of the violations; more frequent status hearings, treatment sessions, or urine tests; and program termination.

Drug courts use various criteria for ending a defendant's participation before completion. These may include a new felony offense, multiple failures to comply with program requirements, and a pattern of positive urine tests. According to the U.S. Department of Justice (1995), many drug courts do not terminate defendants for a new drug possession offense. Before terminating a defendant for continuing to use drugs, drug courts will use an array of treatment services and available sanctions. Similar to other parts of the drug courts' operations, no uniform standards for the number of failed urine tests and failures to attend treatment sessions that result in a participant being terminated apply to all programs. These courts operate with the philosophy that because drug addiction is a disease, relapse can occur, and the court must respond with progressive sanctions and/or enhance treatment rather than immediately terminating a participant. In addition, these programs recognize that some individuals will require a longer period of time to complete the program.

Effectiveness of Drug Courts

The information on the impact of drug courts on recidivism is minimal and mixed. Due to the inherent variety within programs, results of drug court studies must be examined with caution. According to Inciardi, McBride, and Rivers (1996), the most frequently used measure in drug court recidivism studies include (1) felony rearrest rates for both drug and nondrug crimes and (2) time to rearrest. Some studies suggest the original goals for drug courts, reductions in recidivism and drug usage, are being achieved, with recidivism rates substantially reduced for graduates and, to a lesser but significant degree, for participants who do not graduate as well. Drug usage rates for defendants while they are participating in the drug court are also substantially reduced—generally to well under 10 percent, dramatically below that observed for non–drug court offenders (Drug Court Clearinghouse and Technical Assistance Project, 1998). According to a study by American University, recidivism among program graduates runs between 2 and 20 percent, depending upon the characteristics of the population targeted.

In general, less than 3 percent of the recidivism rates for drug court graduates involve violent offenses, and almost all of the small number of violent offenses reported have been misdemeanors. Most of the recidivism reported involves new drug possession charges or traffic violations arising out of driving license suspensions resulting from the initial drug court charge (Drug Court Clearinghouse and Technical Assistance Project, 1998).

Although these evaluations indicate that drug courts may have some beneficial effects, limitations in their design and methodologies, as well as the relative newness of drug courts, preclude firm conclusions about the overall impact of these programs. Other evaluations have shown mixed results in recidivism and other defendant outcomes. For example, a U.S. Department of Justice (1995) document summarizing information about drug courts indicates that two

evaluations showed less recidivism by drug court defendants. However, three other evaluations showed no significant differences in
recidivism. In addition, two evaluations of the same drug court showed
contrasting recidivism results. Also, some studies, such as the research by Brewster (2001), have reported improvements that "approached" but did not meet statistical significance.

Travis County SHORT Program

The current study examines the effect of a drug diversion court in
Austin (Travis County), Texas, on client recidivism. Initiated in August 1993, the Travis County Drug Diversion Court, named the "System of Healthy Options for Release and Transition" or SHORT, is a
one-year, multidisciplinary drug court, case management, and intervention program. The SHORT program became licensed as a supportive outpatient treatment program by the Texas Commission on
Alcohol and Drug Abuse on December 4, 1998.

In general, drug court participants are nonviolent felony offenders
who have been arrested for possession of small amounts of a controlled substance and who are assessed as being addicted to drugs.
The intent of the SHORT program is to break the cycle of drugs and
crime by substituting an effective counseling alternative to traditional
case disposition and incarceration (Travis County Drug Diversion
Court, 1999).

The drug court program operates with a team approach, focuses on
a social service philosophy, closely monitors the progress of each defendant, provides incentives to defendants as appropriate, and admin-
isters graduated sanctions as necessary. Problematic cases are
screened for eligibility by a review committee consisting of a member of the public, law enforcement officers, an assistant district attorney, and court staff.

Participation in the twelve-month SHORT program is voluntary
for eligible defendants and involves deferring prosecution of the defendant's criminal case. In most cases, eligibility for participation is
determined using information gathered by pretrial officers and drug
court intake officers during interviews soon after arrest. After defendants have been deemed eligible, they are educated about the drug
court concept and participate in an orientation that usually occurs
within five days after arrest. Defendants are also required, as a condi-

tion of pretrial release, to participate in an assessment of addiction severity. The participant's first drug court appearance generally takes place within five days after the orientation. During this first appearance, the participant signs a contingency contract with the court. This contract outlines the requirements of the program, including use and frequency of random drug tests; schedule of case-management meetings; sanctions; and payment of fees and court appearances.

The SHORT program operates primarily with a deferred prosecution approach; that is, it targets offenders before their charges have been formally adjudicated. However, some offenders are admitted after their charges have been filed, and in these exceptions, the program takes a postadjudicatory approach. The goal of the SHORT program is to reduce future drug crimes, arrests, and convictions. In addition, the administration has stated the target population to be young African-American males due to the fact that they have been traditionally overrepresented in relation to drug law violations.

The defendant's progression through the SHORT program, like many other drug diversion programs, occurs in three phases, with the individual defendant moving on to each successive phase only after successful completion of the prior phase. Each phase includes frequent urinalysis, drug and alcohol education classes, treatment referrals, and appearances before the drug court judge. At each court appearance, the judge, prosecutor, and defense attorney are provided with up-to-date information on the defendant's progress, recent urinalyses results, and compliance with other program conditions.

Graduate sanctions used in the SHORT program recognize the need to maintain sobriety. Sanctions are used in cases of positive drug test results, lack of satisfactory progress in their individual program, or violations of program rules. A graduated sanctions ladder has been developed to aid the court in assessing "smart punishment" when participants decide to test the limits and boundaries of program rules. Incentives, such as the reduction of program fees or period of supervision, are granted to reward active participation and success in treatment. The ultimate incentive is the dismissal of the defendant's drug charge, without an indictment ever having been filed, upon successful completion of all program requirements (Travis County Drug Diversion Court, 1998).

THE PRESENT STUDY

A random sample of fifty subjects was drawn from a comprehensive list of those individuals admitted to the SHORT program between August 1, 1993, and August 1, 1995. Both computer and manual searches of records were conducted to ensure the entire population of SHORT participants was identified. A control group of fifty individuals was then selected from individuals who were screened for the SHORT program and matched the characteristics of the SHORT participants but who did not attend the SHORT program. The control sample represented individuals who were charged with a felony drug offense during the specified time period but who were denied access to the Travis County Drug Court's SHORT program either by being screened out in the admission process or by refusing the voluntary program.

Subjects in the two samples were matched on the demographic variables of race, gender, age category, employment status at time of arrest, marital status at time of arrest, and previous criminal history (Table 7.1). In addition, all members of both samples were screened by the Travis County Substance Abuse and Counseling Assessment Unit (SACA) and were determined to fit the criteria of "drug dependent" according to their scores on standardized tests. The risk-assessment devices that were used to screen all subjects included the Substance Abuse Subtle Screening Inventory, the Drug Abuse Screening Test, the Mortimer-Filkins Questionnaire, the Michigan Alcohol Screening Test, and the Numerical Drinking Profile (NDP). All scales except the NDP have been shown to be valid and reliable (Mischke & Venneri, 1987; Otto & Hall, 1988; Cocco & Carey, 1998; Rumpf, Hapke, Erfurth, & Johns, 1998). Although the NDP is routinely used by Travis County in screening drug-related cases, no information is readily available as to its development, reliability, or validity. No statistically significant differences were found between the samples based on the demographic variables or drug-dependency variables.

Case outcomes of drug court defendants were compared with the outcomes of the control group defendants. To make sure that the case outcomes were compared in a fair manner, it was necessary to create specific definitions of case outcomes. Since the legal processing of the offenders was different, a single definition of "starting date"

TABLE 7.1. Subject demographics

Demographics	SHORT group (%)	Control group (%)
Race		
Black	36	36
White	56	54
Hispanic	8	10
Gender		
Male	66	64
Female	34	36
Employment status		
Employed	72	76
Unemployed	28	18
Unknown	0	6
Marital status		
Married	18	14
Single	52	48
Divorced	6	10
Widowed	4	0
Other	20	28
Prior criminal history		
None	40	46
Drug/alcohol related	20	18
Nondrug/nonalcohol related	22	20
Both drug and nondrug	18	16

could not be used for all the groups. For SHORT clients, the program starting date was used as a starting point, and for the control group, the date of conviction was used. Outcome measures were taken at three years beyond the starting date for each group. The case outcomes were operationalized in the following manner:

1. *No recidivism*

    SHORT: No arrest and/or convictions after the defendant's date of entry into the program through August 1998

    Control: No arrest and/or conviction after the date of conviction of the initial drug charge which prompted their screening for SHORT through August 1998

2. *Recidivism*

    SHORT: Any arrest and/or conviction after the defendant's date of entry into the program through August 1998

    Control: Any arrest and/or conviction after the date of conviction of the initial drug charge which prompted their screening for SHORT until August 1998

3. *Time to recidivate*

    SHORT: The date of program entry until arrest date was used to measure time to recidivism for clients in the treatment program.

    Control: The date of conviction for the drug offense which prompted each defendant's screening for the SHORT program until arrest date was used to determine time to recidivism for this group.

Demographic, arrest, and conviction data were obtained from the records of Travis County, and recidivism data were verified using TCIC/NCIC (Texas Computerized Information Center/National Crime Information Center).

Definition of Drug- and Alcohol-Related Offenses

The terminology *drug- and/or alcohol-related offenses* within the scope of this study refers to *substance* offenses and includes possession, distribution, or usage of any and all illegal substances, i.e., "possession of a controlled substance," and/or "possession with intent to deliver." Regarding alcohol-related offenses, examples are "driving while intoxicated" or "public intoxication."

Non-drug and/or alcohol offenses refers to all offenses that are not related to the possession, distribution, or usage of any substance, legal or illegal. In this study, whether the individual who committed the criminal act was under the influence of a substance at the time of the commission of the act is not relevant. Crimes are being categorized here, not criminals. For example, if someone was under the influence of an illegal substance while committing an assault, the crime would be categorized under the heading of a non-drug and/or alcohol charge.

MAJOR FINDINGS

Overall recidivism in terms of percentage of arrest and/or convictions for the two groups was as follows. The SHORT clients had thirty-five charges and eighteen convictions. Twenty of the thirty-five charges were drug and/or alcohol related. Ten of the drug- and/or alcohol-related offenses (50 percent) resulted in convictions. For the control group, there were fifty-one charges and thirty-six convictions. Seventy-one percent of all subsequent charges resulted in convictions. Nineteen of the fifty-one charges were drug and/or alcohol related, and fourteen (74 percent) resulted in convictions. See Table 7.2 for a comparison between the two groups.

To examine differences in recidivism between the treatment and control group, a series of t-tests were conducted using the following variables: number of non-drug/alcohol misdemeanor charges, number of non-drug/alcohol felony charges, number of drug/alcohol misdemeanor charges, number of drug/alcohol felony charges, number of non-drug/alcohol misdemeanor convictions, number of non-drug/alcohol felony convictions, number of drug/alcohol misdemeanor convictions, number of drug/alcohol felony convictions, number of months to first charge after initial arrest, and number of months to first conviction after initial arrest. Only statistically significant differences are reported in Table 7.3. The impact of the SHORT program appears to be in its ability to reduce the number of non-drug/alcohol misdemeanor charges. Findings from the study, however, suggest that

TABLE 7.2. Comparison of charges and convictions

Type of offense	SHORT	Control
Drug/alcohol charges	20	19
Drug/alcohol charges convictions	10	14
Non-drug/alcohol charges	5	18
All charges	35	51
All convictions	18	36

TABLE 7.3. Significant differences between the SHORT group and control group

Significant variables	Short mean	Control mean	t-Test significance	Standard error
Non-drug/alcohol-related misdemeanor charges	.18	.44	$P = .044$	.127
Months to first recidivism charge	1.46	4.14	$P = .037$	1.267
Months to first recidivism conviction	1.10	3.68	$P = .036$	1.213

SHORT defendants recidivated more quickly than did their control counterparts, with fewer months from program entry to the first recidivism charge and conviction.

Clearly, as the data demonstrate, the SHORT clients fare no better than do their regular probation counterparts in terms of *overall* recidivism. The SHORT group members were committing similar numbers of drug-related crimes as were the control group members. The fact that the program does appear to reduce the number of non-drug/alcohol misdemeanor charges does not directly fulfill the program objectives of reducing drug-related crime.

There are many explanations as to the causation of these phenomena. One is related to how subjects in the study were assigned to groups. Due to reasons beyond the authors' control, subjects were not able to be randomly assigned to the experimental and control groups. This means that there could be attitudinal differences between the groups that could not be controlled for in this research project. It is possible that characteristics of those individuals who chose to participate in the SHORT program versus those who chose not to participate may have had some effect on their willingness to engage in future criminal behavior. The effect of these possible attitudinal differences is not predictable, but it does require that the results of this study be interpreted with caution.

Another complication in the interpretation of the results of this study is related to the demographic breakdown of the SHORT clientele. The SHORT program states their target population to be young African-American males; however, as indicated by the data, this de-

mographic group is underrepresented in the actual SHORT population. Over half of the SHORT clients were white and about one-third
were female. This issue may affect the ability of the program to demonstrate its effectiveness. It is conceivable to believe that clients who
are female, older, and employed (e.g., nurses who were caught using
prescription drugs), as many of the clients of the program are, have
more incentive to remain out of contact with the criminal justice system than would young, unemployed, poorer clients (Cresswell &
Deschenes, 2001). Since both the SHORT and control groups were
comprised of the same demographics, the program may be at a disad-
vantage in reducing criminal behavior and demonstrating success
with less challenging clients. In effect, both groups had a high "natural" potential for rehabilitation with or without treatment. In a
population with a higher treatment need, a significant difference
might have surfaced.

With respect to the findings that SHORT clients recidivated faster
than control group members, many factors must be examined. One
factor is the manner in which the date considered to be the start point
of measurement for recidivism was selected. For the SHORT group
members, the date they began the program was used as the starting
point to begin measuring recidivism. This was done to ensure that the
treatment being received by the SHORT clients was what could be
considered the source of any differences between groups. For control
group members, the date of conviction for the initial arrest, which resulted in their being screened for the SHORT program, was used as
the starting point for measuring recidivism. This factor may have
contributed to the differences in the number of months it took for
individuals to recidivate.

SUMMARY AND CONCLUSIONS

In the present study, the SHORT clients recidivated almost three
times faster than the control group members. One explanation could
be due to the fact that when SHORT clients were adjudicated to the
SHORT program, they were released back into the community and
had the opportunity to begin recidivating again. It is conceivable that
some of the control group may have remained in custody (jail) during
at least part of the period in which the SHORT clients were already

released. Defendants who have access to private attorneys often gain access to the SHORT program much more quickly and were more likely to be admitted to the program than defendants who have court-appointed attorneys. Second, clients who can afford to make bail and who are released have an advantage in gaining access to the SHORT program. It is possible that defendants who cannot afford to make bail immediately and who have to rely on court-appointed attorneys may have remained in custody for longer periods of time after the initial arrest. The effect of these problems is that some differences in ability to recidivate early may have existed between the groups. The SHORT group may have failed earlier simply because they had access to free-dom faster. It should be noted that the SHORT program staff insti-tuted a new policy of attempting to screen individuals while still in custody shortly after this study was conducted. This would improve the access of individuals who did not make rapid bail to the program.

In addition, with respect to recidivism measurements, a notable problem is the fact that some subsequent charges were grouped with the initial charge when a client completed the program and expunc-tion of records occurred. This is important, because some of the charges that would have been included in the recidivism data were unable to be discovered. In effect, when the SHORT clients had their original offense expunged, some offenses that occurred during their participation in the SHORT program were expunged as well. There-fore, the actual recidivism rate of SHORT clients may have been higher and occurred more rapidly than the results of this research in-dicate. The exact degree of this problem is not known since the re-cords no longer exist as a matter of law. Counselors with the SHORT program are aware that it is happening, but records that indicate how frequently it is happening do not exist.

Another problem faced in the collection of the data for the current study was the fact that SHORT clients were allowed to receive addi-tional charges and convictions, remain in the community, and have additional opportunities to use illegal substances and commit addi-tional criminal acts. The reader should note that in the current study, if the SHORT client did not succeed in getting an expunction order, these charges and convictions were tabulated in the recidivism data. This is an important difference between the operation of the SHORT program and offenders in the control group who were on regular pro-bation. When a defendant on regular probation is arrested and convicted for a subsequent offense, probation is typically revoked, and the offender is incarcerated to serve time for the original charge for which he or she was convicted. The nature of the drug court's philosophy in presuming that SHORT clients are prone to relapse due to their addiction gave offenders the chance to get more than one additional charge before any action was taken. This could have had an upward bias in the data on new charges for the SHORT clients.

Specifically, for the Travis County Drug Diversion Court, it is imperative that replication studies of this research be conducted in order to gain deeper insight into the recidivism of SHORT clients. Measures of client recidivism, which would allow the tracking of data such as expunged offenses, need to be developed and utilized in program evaluation. In addition, careful consideration needs to be given to the demographics of offenders admitted to the program to ensure that they match the population for which the program is designed (Miller & Shutt, 2001). As discussed earlier, clients who are conducive to rehabilitation, such as middle-aged white females with careers, are being admitted in place of clients who would most likely be more difficult to rehabilitate. While the creaming of clients can make simple descriptive data look good, the effects are neutralized when the clients are compared to a suitable control group. In the case of this particular research, creaming of clients may be one of the reasons that the evaluation was unable to demonstrate client success. Since federal funding for the program is based on the program's ability to show effectiveness in reducing drug-related criminal behavior, it is critical that better outcome measures and client screening be implemented.

Due to the amount of financial support and resources being directed toward drug courts, it is important to continue conducting research on their overall effectiveness. Until uniform standards of both the operation and the evaluation of drug diversion courts are developed and followed, the results of recidivism studies will continue to be largely descriptive and useless in terms of generalization. Training in the methods of scientific research for drug court administrators and staff members involved in the reporting of drug court effectiveness should also be implemented.

Suggestions for future drug court administrators and the national drug court community involve the standardization of program operations, treatment, funding, evaluation, and the ability to create a more controlled program environment which would provide more knowledge about the offender's actual behavior in the program. Some may view drug court programs as too lenient a punishment for the drug offender. Others may argue that the treatment focus of the drug court is the most important concern. More careful monitoring of the client in the community can help satisfy both of these interests. This should both increase community safety and enhance treatment effectiveness.

DISCUSSION QUESTIONS

1. How would you describe the basic components of drug courts? What are the specific criteria and goals of the Travis County drug court as described by Cunningham and Stone?
2. What were some of the major differences between the authors' control group and experimental group when it comes to recidivism among drug court clientele?
3. Discuss the possible explanations, as discussed by Cunningham and Stone, for these findings.
4. In light of these findings, what suggestions do they make for future research in this area and for the placement of clients in this type of programming?

REFERENCES

Brewster, M. (2001). Evaluation of the Chester County (PA) drug court program. *Journal of Drug Issues, 31*(1), 177-206.

Cocco, K. & Carey, K. (1998). Psychometric properties of the Drug Abuse Screening Test in psychiatric outpatients. *Psychological Assessment, 10*(4), 408-414.

Cresswell, L. & Deschenes, E. (2001). Minority and non-minority perceptions of drug court program severity and effectiveness. *Journal of Drug Issues, 31*(1), 259-292.

Drug Court Clearinghouse and Technical Assistance Project. (1998). Looking at a decade of drug courts. Available at <www.ncjrs.org/html/bja/decade98.htm>.

Federal Bureau of Investigation. (2000). *Uniform crime reports 1999*. Washington, DC: U.S. Department of Justice.

Inciardi, J., McBride, C., & Rivers, J. (1996). *Drug control and the courts: Drugs, health, and social policy series* (Vol. 3). Thousand Oaks, CA: Sage.

Miller, M. & Shutt, E. (2001). Considering the need for empirically grounded drug court screening mechanisms. *Journal of Drug Issues, 31*(1), 91-106.

Mischke, H. & Venneri, R. (1987). Reliability and validity of the MAST, Mortimer-Filkins and CAGE in DWI assessment. *Journal of Studies on Alcohol, 48,* 492-501.

Otto, R. & Hall, J. (1988). The utility of the Michigan Alcoholism Screening Test in the detection of alcoholism and problem drinkers. *Journal of Personality Assessment, 52,* 499-505.

Rumpf, H., Hapke, U., Erfurth, A., & John, U. (1998). Screening questionnaires in the detection of hazardous alcohol consumption in the general hospital: Direct or disguised assessment? *Journal of Studies on Alcohol, 59*(6), 698-703.

Travis County Drug Diversion Court. (1999). Available at <www.co.travis.tx.us/district_courts/drug_courts>.

Turque, B. (1989, May 29). Why can't justice be done: America's courts and prisons are overwhelmed. *Newsweek,* pp. 36-37.

U.S. Department of Justice. (1995). Drug courts: Proposed rule. Available at <www.druglibrary.org/schaffer/GovPubs/DRUGCRT.HTM>.

Chapter 8

Setting the Stage for Treating Drug Court Clients: How to Initiate Treatment

Robert Walker
TK Logan

The overall purpose of this chapter is to provide substance abuse counselors with information on how to begin substance abuse treatment with drug court clients. This chapter will include information about how to initiate treatment with adult drug court clients and how to establish clear communications and relationships among clients, counselors, and the court. In addition, the chapter will include recommendations for appropriate methods of communicating to the court about drug court client progress.

Recognizing the difficulty in working with court-referred clients, this chapter focuses on the critical pretreatment processes that can contribute to more successful treatment. Pretreatment processes, such as informing clients clearly about service limitations and providing detailed informed consent, can influence how treatment is perceived and delivered. With careful attention to informed consent and the setting of an appropriate context for counseling court-referred clients, treatment has a better chance of promoting constructive change. With careful application of pretreatment processes that define the context of counseling, less-structured clinical approaches such as motivational interviewing may be used with greater fidelity.

There is great need for more research on effective treatment approaches with court-referred and substance-abusing clients with antisocial traits (Marlowe et al., 2001). In addition, there is only a very limited literature on pretreatment issues (Leukefeld, Tims, & Platt,

2001). This chapter draws from the literature and makes recommendations on how to initiate treatment to make the most productive use of interventions.

The use of motivational approaches (Miller & Rollnick, 1991, 2002) has been examined for court-referred clients (Ginsburg, Mann, Rotgers, & Weekes, 2002). However, there is an innate tension between the client-friendly nature of motivational interviewing and the constraints of court-mandated treatment (Ginsburg et al., 2002). The careful use of pretreatment definition of services, roles, the limits on confidentiality, the risks and benefits of treatment, and informed consent to treatment can greatly enhance the application of motivational approaches. The constraints involved with court-referred counseling are discussed prior to client participation, and clients act as free agents in agreeing to treatment within these constraints. Informed consent, which includes providing clients with sufficient information to make decisions about their health and well-being, addresses client autonomy and has important applications to treatment for behavioral disorders (Beahrs & Gutheil, 2001; Berg, Appelbaum, Lidz, & Parker, 2001; Faden & Beauchamp, 1999).

The pretreatment counseling approaches described in this chapter supplement publications by the Substance Abuse and Mental Health Services Administration (SAMHSA) and the Center for Substance Abuse Treatment (CSAT) such as "Treatment Drug Courts: Integrating Substance Abuse Treatment with Legal Case Processing" (Sherin & Mahoney, 1996) and "Substance Abuse Treatment Planning Guide and Checklist for Treatment-Based Drug Courts" (CSAT, 1997). These publications describe ways to establish effective relationships between treatment and drug court programs and include basic components of treatment programs for drug court clients. In contrast to these publications, this chapter describes specific clinical approaches that counselors can use to facilitate the initiation of treatment.

By way of introduction, it is important to recognize that treatment is but one component of clients' participation in drug court. The court may not view treatment as the critical component in client participation in drug court. Other areas, such as employment, education, and client compliance with other court requirements, may take precedence over counseling about drug problems. Counselors should recognize the relative importance of treatment in clients' participation in drug courts and set expectations accordingly. They should also recognize that clients must meet graduated levels of responsibility at different phases of participation. Counseling and treatment should be compatible with the phased structure of the drug court program. For example, clients enter drug courts under very close supervision. The initiation of treatment generally takes place when the supervisory process is most intense. The initiation of counseling should reflect this greater emphasis on close supervision and vigilance about engagement with treatment. In all phases of drug court, clients face sanctions for resumed use of illicit substances and/or alcohol. With this in mind, treatment should adopt an abstinence goal in all drug court phases but should be particularly clear about this goal during the initiation of treatment. It is important to note that an abstinence goal is not the same as an insistence on abstinent behavior. Counselors can adopt an abstinence coaching role that promotes the goals of drug court while at the same time encourages incremental change and growth. The abstinence coaching role can be helpful during the initiation into drug court treatment since it communicates a willingness to work with clients toward improvement rather than just policing compliance.

This chapter also describes pretreatment that is contextualized to drug court clients' criminal lifestyle or personality along with their substance abuse. Having been charged with criminal offenses, there is a likelihood of criminal thought patterns that guide client behaviors (Yochelson & Samenow, 1976, 1977). Rather than separating the two behavioral issues, this chapter assumes an integrated approach that incorporates simultaneous attention to criminal thinking and substance abuse. This is why these pretreatment approaches define clear limits to counselor roles as well as very clear limits on confidentiality and the opportunities for manipulative communications by clients.

In one sense, drug court clients might be compared to dual-diagnosis clients in that they have two overlapping and interacting problems: substance abuse and criminal thinking and behaving. Research suggests that the two disorders often co-occur (van den Bree, Svikis, & Pickens, 2000). Successful treatment should address both conditions in an integrated way since both conditions interact in self-defeating ways (Walker, 1992a,b; Wanberg & Milkman, 1998). The two conditions co-occur at very high rates. In fact, the co-occurrence of substance abuse and criminality is such that the overwhelming majority of prisoners are drug users (Leukefeld & Tims, 1992; Leukefeld, Tims, & Farabee, 2002). Since many drug court clients have antisocial or criminal personality traits, the initiation of treatment must be particularly sensitive to criminal thought processes and the need for counselors to be truthful about every aspect of treatment (Yochelson & Samenow, 1977).

Some substance abuse counselors prefer not to work with drug court clients because of clients' quasi-involuntary status and counselors' beliefs that court-referred clients do not do well in treatment. The clinical approaches described in this chapter were developed using available research on client characteristics and the clinical literature focused on court-referred clients with criminal thinking patterns. Criminal thinking–focused approaches are supported in the clinical literature. This approach is also grounded in research on court-referred, antisocial client characteristics (Fishbein, 2000; Raine, 1994).

Research has also consistently shown that clients who are referred from the criminal justice system do as well or better than other "voluntary" clients (Polcin, 2001; Farabee, Prendergast, & Anglin, 1998; Anglin & Hser, 1991). In fact, court-ordered treatment for substance abuse has been found to have better outcomes than voluntary treatment (Donovan & Rosengren, 1999; Leukefeld et al., 2002). Furthermore, drug courts have been shown to be effective in reducing drug use among offenders and in reducing social and financial costs to society (Logan et al., in press). Some studies report that drug court graduates do better than a control group after leaving the program, and this finding is consistent with previous research (Belenko 1999, 2001). However, not all studies report the same differences between graduates and control groups (Belenko, 1999, 2001).

Given evidence of the positive outcomes from drug court participation, it is important to provide more information about the treatment aspect of drug court and how it can be improved. One of the aims of this chapter is to help counselors establish more successful clinical relationships with drug court clients and thus provide treatment with a greater likelihood of positive outcomes.

KEY COMPONENTS OF DRUG COURTS

Counselors working with drug court clients must have a clear understanding of the basic structure and policies of drug courts. Drug courts vary from jurisdiction to jurisdiction, but most share in implementing ten key components, which serve as both guiding principles and core service elements. The ten components reflect the integration of treatment with criminal justice supervision and sanctioning, and treatment does not stand apart from the overall supervision and sanctioning processes. Drug courts generally include the following components or criteria (U.S. Department of Justice, 1997; Belenko, 1999, 2002; Drug Courts Program Office, 1997):

1. Drug courts integrate alcohol and other drug treatment services with justice system case processing.
2. Using a nonadversarial approach, prosecution and defense counsel promote public safety while protecting participants' due process right.
3. Eligible participants are indentified early and promptly placed in the drug court program.
4. Drug courts provide access to a continuum of alcohol and other drug testing.
5. Abstinence is monitored by frequent alcohol and other drug testing.
6. A coordinated strategy governs drug court responses to participants' compliance.
7. Ongoing judicial interaction with each drug court participant is essential.
8. Monitoring and evaluation measure the achievement of program goals and gauge effectiveness.
9. Continuing interdisciplinary education promotes effective drug court planning, implementation, and operations.
10. Forging partnerships among drug courts, public agencies, and community-based organizations generates local support and enhances drug court effectiveness.

Drug court clients must meet basic admission criteria including a history of substance abuse. Clients with a history of violent offenses or clients who are found to be drug dealers without substance abuse problems are generally not eligible for admission. Admission to drug courts can occur under probation terms or diversion where records are expunged after successful treatment. Participants sign an agreement to participate with an understanding of the requirements of the program including providing urine specimens, attending treatment, and complying with other program stipulations if accepted into the drug court program. It takes, on average, eighteen to twenty-four months for participants to successfully graduate. Graduation generally means that clients have completed program requirements and have had clean results from their drug tests over a sustained period of time (Logan, Williams, & Leukefeld, 2001). Although clients with known histories of violent charges are generally not accepted into drug courts, counselors should understand that given the associations of violence with substance use, it is likely that drug court clients may present histories of violence, including domestic violence, since substance abuse is prevalent among almost half of domestic violence offenders (Holtzworth-Munroe, Smultzler, & Sandin, 1997).

FOUNDATION FOR UNDERSTANDING SUBSTANCE ABUSE AND CRIME

The following points of view can be important for counselors in initiating treatment for drug court clients. Having an overall working theory about the relationship between substance abuse and crime can be important for counselors as well as drug court staff. Counselors are encouraged to have a basic operating theory of the interaction between criminality and substance use that can help guide their clinical interactions with drug court clients. Although there are no easy explanations for the co-occurrence of these two problem areas, there are several basic ways to understand the following possible relationships between the two.

> *Drug use leads to crime:* For some clients, criminal conduct has emerged as a result of becoming drug or alcohol involved. The costs of increasing drug or alcohol use, coupled with the illegality of most substances, can explain a person's evolution into progressively more criminal conduct. As a person associates more and more with illicit drug suppliers and other users, criminal conduct becomes more a part of the lifestyle. In these cases, the person is socialized into crime as a result of drug/alcohol use.
>
> *Crime leads to drug use:* A person who is engaged in crime is exposed to drug use since drug use is so prevalent in the criminal culture. Criminal lifestyles include drug use, and with exposure to substances there is always a risk of becoming de-

pendent or a substance abuser. This group might also be seen as being socialized into drug use just as some drug users are socialized into criminal behavior.

Criminal personality traits predispose some individuals to drug use: There are some drug-involved persons with criminality whose criminal conduct emerged in early childhood. For these persons, drug use appears to be but one aspect of their overall criminal traits. High impulsivity, risk-taking behavior, sensation seeking, lack of remorse, and early manifestation of overt criminal behavior such as theft while confronting a person, use of weapons, or sexual assault can be a part of this set of traits. In these cases, drug use is a part of the overall antisocial personality.

Mental and emotional problems result in drug use: Some persons with mood disorders such as depression or with anxiety disorders can begin using drugs and alcohol to medicate their emotional problems. There is considerable research on substance abuse by victims of trauma who experience depression and anxiety disorders such as post-traumatic stress disorder (PTSD). Likewise, while pain-management authorities disagree with the idea that persons can become addicted to narcotic analgesics as a result of medication for authentic pain, some persons might abuse legitimate prescriptions to the point of becoming heavily drug involved. This group might be understood as self-medicating emotional or physical symptoms.

Poverty and lifestyle cause drug use: Low-income communities may offer limited reward experiences for people. Youth, in particular, may be vulnerable to the need to find some avenue for relief from despair and the depressing situations in which they live. Likewise, they may seek pleasurable experiences with their peers in one of the few ways that are available in inner cities or very rural areas—drug and alcohol use. Although poverty may be a risk factor for substance abuse and criminal activity, it is not directly causal since there are many more people in poverty who are not substance abusers or criminals.

The traditional explanations of substance abuse and dependence are often implicit in the treatment approaches used by counselors. For example, counselors who believe that substance dependence is at the heart of criminal conduct will *treat the drug problem* and believe that this approach resolves the criminal problems as well. Counselors who focus mostly on personality disorders might *treat the underlying antisocial or borderline personality* structure and believe that drug use will decrease as self-destructive personality traits are modified. The current understanding of addiction as a disease process (Leshner, 1997) does not lessen the importance of understanding the role of other disorders along with substance use disorders. This is critical with drug court clients in which there is extensive co-occurrence of drug use and criminality such that treatment must simultaneously focus on both conditions—the drug use *and* the criminal behavior *irrespective of the cause/effect relationship between the two conditions.*

THE COUNSELOR-CLIENT RELATIONSHIP

It is critical to understand that the counselor-client relationship in drug court cases is different from traditional counselor-client relationships. For drug court cases, the relationship is best understood as a triangle. As illustrated in Figure 8.1, the triangle is a three-C construct: the court-client-counselor relationship. The successful initiation of treatment depends on a careful description of the "three Cs," and all three parties must understand this arrangement. Traditional mental health and substance abuse professionals' ethical construction of counselor-client relationships have focused on a dyad and the importance of keeping third parties remote from the all-important confidentiality dimension. However, the social construction of drug court treatment imposes a modification of this traditional dyadic relationship. In fact, it is in clients' best interests to have clear communication

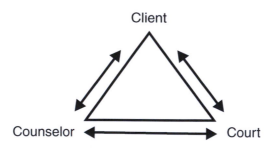

FIGURE 8.1. The court-client-counselor relationship in drug court cases

among all parties from the very beginning of treatment. Clients must be made aware of the significant limitations on traditional confidentiality in these referral situations. When counselors fail to clarify these communication issues at the very beginning of treatment, there is the likelihood of problems later in treatment when clients are shocked to see the results of counselor communications with the court. Attention to the triangular relationship at the beginning of treatment also conveys truthfulness about the benefits and constraints of court-referred treatment. Declaring the limitations on confidentiality *before* the client gives permission for treatment fulfills a true informed consent process about proceeding with treatment. This means that there is a clear exchange between all three parties. The counselor should get information from the drug court as well as from the client. Likewise, the counselor will inform the drug court about client progress.

Communication is crucial to the drug court treatment process. When only two of the three enter into communication, it means that one party is left in a difficult position. If it is clients who are in the dark, then it is likely that at some point clients will discover or infer a "deal" between the counselor and the drug court. A perception of this kind of "deal" between the professionals can contribute to clients' negative view of treatment. This situation can also validate the criminal view of authorities as untruthful, untrustworthy, and manipulative. These projections can be substantiated when counselors are not, in fact, truthful. The net effect can be a validation of the very criminal thought processes that are the subject of treatment.

If counselors are left out of important communications between clients and the drug court staff, counselors will feel disempowered to be of any help to clients. In this situation, counselors will generally withdraw interest from the counseling and will do the minimum necessary to meet agency obligations. This is an unfortunate outcome for clients, counselors, and drug court staff since it means the dismissal of the possibility of change through the counseling process.

If the court is excluded from important communications between counselors and clients, then counselors can be seen as colluding with clients against the court. When counselors give clients permission to miss sessions or to avoid required tasks, it can suggest to the court that counselors have simply been conned. If counselors are easily conned by clients, they will have very little credibility with the drug court and potentially with the judge and other court personnel. This situation can lead to a disrespectful attitude toward treatment and treatment providers.

MANAGING THE PRETREATMENT CONTEXT FOR COUNSELING

The initiation of treatment is perhaps the most important part of treatment with drug court clients. A well-prepared clinical setting for counseling can prevent many of the impasses and conflicts that can arise when both counselor and client "stumble" into successive situations during treatment. With this in mind, counselors should pay close attention to several professional functions that should take place before treatment or counseling begin.

Counseling with drug court clients often means frequent encounters with denial. It is so prevalent that counselors should expect denial both of substance abuse and related problems. The very earliest phases of treatment can be distorted by prevalent denial if counselors take it literally. However, if counselors understand that denial is an opening move on a chessboard and that drug court clients are attempting to take control of one small area of life, then the experience can be viewed differently. There are three important components in managing the pretreatment context for counseling: (1) obtaining relevant referral information; (2) providing the client with pertinent pretreatment information; and (3) setting a constructive frame of reference for treatment.

Obtaining Relevant Referral Information

Counselors should obtain official background referral information from the drug court *before* beginning intake interviews. This is important for structuring the interview as well as demonstrating the level of communications between counselors and the drug court. As described previously, the counseling situation involves a triangular relationship between the counselors, clients, and the court. If counselors learn about clients' referral circumstances from clients rather than from the drug court, it puts the client in the role of controlling and shaping the "spin" on referral information that the counselor receives. Counselors need to have the "official" version of clients' referral situation before hearing clients' view of their court involvement.

This does not mean that clients' views are wrong or that they should be dismissed. The problem with hearing about referral conditions from clients is that the power structure of the relationship is disturbed by this approach.

Counselors should hear and appreciate clients' view of the referral situation, but the "official" referral information should come from the drug court. This way, clients' charges, drug court phase assignments, and other relevant information can be related directly to the counselor. The ethics of counseling are better served when the drug court makes the referral and informs the counselor of the court referral. This way, an open triangular relationship can be assertively identified for clients. In the absence of a formal referral from the drug court, the counselor has an ethical duty only to the individual client. The introduction of the drug court into the equation after treatment has begun is ethically more ambiguous and is more likely to result in problems in the therapeutic relationship between the counselor and client. Intake should be grounded in the drug court referral information, and clients should be informed that this information has been provided to facilitate the intake process.

Pretreatment Information Provided to Clients About Treatment

Once referral information has been obtained from the drug court, counselors can provide clients with pretreatment information *before intake/assessment interviews begin*. The initial contact with clients should include attention to several pretreatment information issues. The following pretreatment guidelines are recommended before formal intake/assessment interviews begin. It is important for counselors to provide this pretreatment information to clients in a friendly, matter-of-fact way. This approach is recommended as an alternative to presenting rigid "program rules." The intent of these pretreatment guidelines is to make the counseling situation honest and realistic and to reduce inaccurate views of what counseling and treatment are going to involve. By setting the stage for all the clinical interactions, counselors can reduce their problems with uncooperative responses later on in treatment. These *pretreatment approaches* establish a working contract between counselors and clients and minimize the likelihood of misunderstandings later in treatment. These initial procedures are also designed to reduce the effects and manipulative aspects of denial throughout the intake process.

1. Counselors should begin with an appreciation for clients' follow-through with the appointments. Drug court clients receive little positive feedback for their constructive and responsible actions. Counselors should highlight everything positive that clients do even if it includes small matters such as keeping appointments. Keeping an appointment should never be taken for granted. The initial contacts with treatment staff should include a positive, strengths-enhancing approach that builds on what the client does well.

2. Counselors should obtain clients' permission for assessment and treatment services and include the following information as part of the process for obtaining informed consent to treatment:

- Informed consent includes information about the *risks and benefits* of treatment much as operative consent forms describe the possible risks that can occur with surgery. Clients should understand that counseling involves not only the possibilities of positive change but also uncovering unpleasant memories and emotions, as well as possible risks from nonattendance in treatment.
- There are clear risks to participation in substance abuse treatment including a *risk of reincarceration or other sanctions* for failure to participate in treatment.
- There is *very limited confidentiality* under drug court referral situations. Clients should understand the triangular communication relationships that exist in this type of treatment setting and the limits on confidentiality as a risk of treatment since disclosed information can result in further disclosure to the court with a potential for unwanted consequences.
- *Client commitments* to treatment should be discussed, including fees, time commitments for group and individual sessions, and the anticipated duration of treatment.

3. Counselors should explain that the informed consent information is a *protection of client rights and personal well-being*—not merely a set of required procedures. In other words, clients should be provided with this information as a service, not a mere bureaucratic requirement.

4. Counselors should explain their responsibility to *report clients' treatment progress* to the court. It is important to tell clients that counselors must make routine reports to the drug court and what those reports typically contain. Clients should be made aware of these reports at the very beginning of treatment.

5. Counselors should explain that they are *not attorneys or advocates* and that it is not a counselor's role to represent clients or take clients' side in an adversarial way in the drug court process. Although counselors may, in fact, assist clients in dealing with inequities in the system once they are in treatment, this should not be presented during the initiation of treatment. Counselors should avoid overt advocacy except in situations where clients have demonstrated their reliability and undistorted representation of events—factors that cannot be in evidence during intake.

6. Counselors should explain that clients, in signing the permission for treatment, also must give counselors authorization to communicate with the court. The new federal Health Insurance Portability and Accountability Act (HIPAA) requirements governing protected health information may be in place with drug court treatment. These new requirements provide additional protections for personal health information. Substance abuse treatment providers and counselors must determine whether they are "covered entities" under the HIPAA regulations. If they are deemed covered entities, separate client authorizations for using and disclosing protected health information must be used. In addition, counselors who are independent of the drug court may have to enter into "business associate agreements" with drug courts in order to use drug court client information. The permission for treatment should either include an authorization for release of information or, if HIPAA regulations apply, should reference that the permission for treatment is contingent on a separate authorization to release information. The permission for treatment should also state that in the absence of an authorization to release information, the permission for treatment will be considered revoked and continued services cannot be provided without permission for treatment. This means that clients who refuse to permit release of information cannot continue to be provided with counseling under the current referral context.

7. Counselors should *explain the scope of services* and specific areas of client needs that can be addressed such as mental health prob-

lems or employment-related needs (Walker & Leukefeld, 2002), as well as trauma-related service needs which have been identified as extensive among substance-using women in particular (Logan, Walker, Cole, & Leukefeld, 2002).

8. Counselors should explain the *legal duties to report* child abuse, domestic violence, or threats to harm others and the duties to hospitalize clients who are suicidal or who have serious mental illness and who pose an immediate threat to others.

9. Counselors should explain that counselors and treatment centers can *work only with persons who have a substance use problem* and that if a client has absolutely *no* problem, then admission to the program is impossible. (This should be done in a matter-of-fact manner. It is simply a statement, not an effort at persuading a client to "get on board.") This step may be important even for those who wish to use motivational interviewing approaches once treatment has begun. The information provides a background for seeking client direction in treatment while at the same time provides a fallback for counselors when clients deny any drug-related problems.

10. Counselors should assess clients' understanding of these principles. Counselors should ask clients to sign a *permission for treatment* form after these pretreatment issues have been discussed. If a client refuses to sign a permission for treatment, counselors should inform the client that the counseling session cannot be provided without the permission being signed. The counselor should offer the client an opportunity to reconsider. If the client still does not want to sign a permission for treatment form, then the session should be terminated politely and the client should be informed that the counselor will send a letter to the drug court stating "Mr. John Doe was scheduled for an assessment session on [date]. Mr. Doe did not sign a permission for treatment and thus services could not be provided. Should he wish to return and sign a permission for treatment, counseling services will be provided." This approach keeps the door open to reconsideration after further discussions between the drug court staff and the client. This approach also keeps the counselor out of the position of trying to talk the client into treatment—an approach that can distort the proper relationship between a counselor and client. At no point in these discussions should counselors appear angry or upset with a client decision not to sign a permission for treatment. The counselor stance should be friendly, cooperative, and understanding of clients' per-

spectives. The drug court staff should be the "enforcers" or persuaders for treatment.

Setting the Clinical Frame of Reference

The best starting point for counseling, as stated earlier, is to inform clients that the program only serves persons who have a drug or alcohol problem. This approach sets a *clinical frame of reference* that can be referred to throughout treatment. For example, if a client begins to deny any drug problem five weeks into treatment, the counselor can remind the client that the agency can schedule appointments only with those who in fact have problems to work on. Not having a problem may mean that the client's services will terminated. Some counselors try to work with drug court clients using standard interview approaches that assume internal motivations to seek help. On not seeing evidence of these motivations, counselors may find themselves trying to persuade clients that they really do have problems and that they need treatment even though the client denies everything. In these situations, counselors can become frustrated by feeling that the client controls the sessions by withholding participation.

One way to avoid this dilemma is to set a different frame of reference for counseling. By informing clients that counselors make appointments only for clients who have problems, the burden of proof shifts away from counselors and back to clients to justify why they are applying for services. Simple analogies can illustrate this point for clients. Counselors can compare the interview situation to a person going to see a dentist because a family member "told him" to go. In this example, when the patient gets in the dentist's chair, he says he has "no problem" and will not open his mouth. Counselors can ask clients, "What would the dentist do next after explaining that it was important to have one's teeth examined?" "Would the dentist spend two or three sessions trying to *convince the patient* about the need to agree that there is a dental problem that needs treatment?" "Is a dentist likely to spend a lot of time trying to plead with a patient to open his mouth when there are other people waiting for services?" The case should be presented in a lighthearted and even humorous way to illustrate the point about the availability of counseling services. Counselors should explain this as a circumstance beyond counselors' control so as to not portray it as a personal matter—simply a factor that is applied to all clients.

The purpose of clear and business-like discussions at the beginning of services is to establish trust and honest transactions. Counselors should not sugarcoat treatment or program expectations when serving drug court clients. Instead, a kind and receptive but firm manner is advised. Discussing risks at the very outset is a way of making "the system's" rules open and above board. It reduces the likelihood of a surprise about reports to the drug court when clients fail to meet treatment expectations. It is also important for counselors to be extremely honest with drug court clients because of the nature of criminal thinking patterns. Many court-involved clients have well-established patterns of lying. Drug court clients also expect others to lie and use this belief to justify their own deceptions. Counselors can accidentally fall into a trap when they are not fully open with clients about requirements for reporting to the court, for following abuse report laws, or about setting treatment expectations. Treatment stands a better chance of success if counselors discuss all the hard facts with clients before treatment has begun.

Issues Related to Communication with the Court

As mentioned previously, the permission for treatment should be linked with an authorization to release information to the court. This is similar to other treatment procedure permits. Surgery, for example, requires anesthesia, which has its own level of risk above and beyond the risks due to surgery. The operative consent form informs patients that one cannot have the surgery without the anesthesia. Since drug court substance abuse treatment cannot be practiced without a counselor being able to communicate with the court, the release of information is an essential aspect of the treatment approach. *Counselors cannot provide counseling effectively or correctly with drug court clients without open communication with the drug court or other court personnel.* To begin treatment without this type of linked permission for treatment/release of information has a risk of setting the stage for client manipulation of counselors. If counselors provide services without a release of information that is linked to the permission for treatment, counselors can appear to be in collusion with clients since the communications with the drug court would be cut off even though treatment may continue. In these situations, clients can exercise unconstructive control over the counseling service and defeat the goal of treating criminal thinking.

Although counselors need to report client progress to the drug court, this communication does not need to include more than the necessary and minimum information. Clients should be informed about the type of information that will be communicated to the court. Letters should not include any "spin" or hint of counselors' feeling about clients. For example, the first letter to a drug court after a client assessment should contain the following information:

- The client name, date of the assessment interview, and place where the interview occurred
- A statement about the client's problem, i.e., "Mr. Doe reports cocaine use."
- A preliminary treatment plan such as "weekly individual counseling appointments and weekly group therapy sessions for the next twelve weeks"
- A report of the client's agreement to participate, such as "Mr. Doe has agreed to attend the weekly individual and group sessions."

Drug court reports need not include extensive personal information. In fact, this practice is not recommended. Counselors' assessment reports and routine reports to the drug court should be brief as well. The letters also should refer to clients as "Mr.," "Ms.," or "Mrs." The use of first names can suggest a degree of familiarity that can be inappropriate. These letters should include a statement of attendance (preferably actual dates of attendance) and a brief statement about progress or degree of participation. A letter might include a statement such as "Mr. Doe has kept three of four individual appointments [date], [date], and [date]. He has been active in the group sessions and has participated in individual sessions as well." Counselors should provide clients with sample letters to show the type of information that is likely to be included in communications about them.

Counselors should not use judgment-laden language in making reports to the drug court. Noncompliant clients can elicit anger and frustration among counselors. Letters and reports to the drug court should report facts, not opinions that give evidence of counselors' negative feelings about clients. *Terms such as "resistance," "unmoti-*

vated," and "manipulative" should be avoided since they can convey a personal dislike or biased feeling toward clients. Instead, counselors should report facts and let the court make judgments about the behavior. For example, instead of describing a client as "resistive," the counselor could state that "the client has not spoken during group sessions and has volunteered no personal information."

Special Considerations: Culture, Gender, Ethnicity

Cultural, gender, racial, and ethnic factors should be considered in initiating treatment. Cultural competency has become a standard for most substance abuse treatment programs. Accreditation organizations have also incorporated cultural competency as a standard. It is included as an ethical issue for many professionals who are licensed or certified. Although cultural competency has become a critical issue in treatment, there is little guidance on how to assess or build cultural competence. Specialized cultural diversity training programs have a difficult time avoiding promotion of stereotypes in spite of a desire to avoid stereotyping (Walker & Staton, 2000).

It is critical for counselors to have a clear understanding of clients' cultural background and how it shapes attitudes, values, and behaviors and can color their understanding of the terms of treatment. It is equally important for counselors to be aware of their own culture and how it affects the counselor's understanding of clients at the beginning of treatment. There is no easy way to assess the degree to which counselors can misunderstand client cultural factors. However, when counselors become overly judgmental about "unmotivated" clients or too eager for drug court sanctions, this can provide a cue that cultural understanding is missing. Likewise, counselors may have a naive understanding of clients, and this can be related to difficulty in understanding and relating appropriately to different cultures.

Counselors who have empathy and compassion for their clients will approach clients with cultural sensitivity and without labels or stereotypes that can be harmful. Unfortunately, empathy and compassion are not skills that can be easily taught. Counselors' introspection may be helpful in addressing cultural factors as well. Supervisors can be helpful in calling problems to the attention of counselors. Many instances of cultural insensitivity result from a lack of awareness. Problem awareness is an important step toward solution. Most counselors want to help clients, but cultural blindness can make this difficult. Treatment staff who share clients' culture may be helpful in stimulating discussion about cultural differences and their meaning in counseling.

Gender issues are also critical variables in the treatment of substance abuse clients. While most drug court clients are male, female clients are also referred for treatment. Victimization is a significant problem for many women in substance abuse treatment. A recent review of the literature points to complex interactions between substance abuse and victimization in women (Logan et al., 2002). Logan et al.'s (2002) review of the literature suggests that about 80 percent of female clients in substance abuse treatment have interpersonal abuse histories. The initiation of treatment with women should involve a focus on victimization that includes permission to raise victimization issues as well as addressing safety planning. The recovery process from substance abuse, when coupled with childhood abuse, can be slow and marked by many complications with drug-using women. However, while drug court treatment is a coercive process, it is important to not coerce female clients into disclosure of abuse issues unless the client wants to pursue them (Herman, 1992). Coercion can evoke negative feelings about power and control among victims that have nothing to do with resistance to treatment or denial of substance abuse problems. The reactions may arise from abuse experiences. The use of sanctions can reinforce a client's sense of loss of control over her own life and personal history. In general, if the victimization issues are the dominant concern, then a referral to a domestic violence victims' program may be a more appropriate first step in treatment. Counselors should assess whether the substance abuse levels are stable enough for a victimization focus or whether substance abuse recovery must be targeted before the victimization. Finally, sensitivity to gender issues may mean that treatment should be provided by female counselors—particularly given the coercive elements involved in drug court treatment.

SUMMARY AND CONCLUSIONS

Although drug courts have been found to have positive treatment outcomes among substance abusers, there are many complexities in providing treatment under court-referred circumstances. If, for example, drug court programs are going to work to bring down both substance abuse and crime, both the court and the counselors must recognize that these two problems cannot be separated from each other. Just as treatment in noncorrectional settings moves toward the realization that most substance abusers copresent with other problems as well, problems that must be addressed concurrently with substance abuse treatment, correctional managers/administrators should consider moving in a similar direction. Regardless of the temporal order of the relationship between substance abuse and crime, the evidence suggests that the two are related. To treat one while ignoring the other sets up a program for possible failure.

Closer attention to the pretreatment issues such as defining services carefully, establishing boundaries, and obtaining authentic informed consent may help reduce resistance and misunderstandings between counselors and clients. Programs that do not make it clear up front that the counselor must report information gained from sessions to the drug court risk turning off clients and the possibility of losing them. Although there is a fine line between reporting requirements and clients feeling comfortable enough to actively participate in treatment, effective treatment under these circumstances can be achieved through careful and deliberate steps taken by the counselor.

Substance abuse treatment for drug court clients may depend on careful attention to pretreatment issues at the initiation of services. Given the importance of the helping relationship between the drug court client and his or her counselor, it may be critical to set an appropriate frame for treatment that gives clients reasonable expectations of the possible outcomes of participation as well as risks that can be involved. Hopefully the information presented here will assist practitioners, and drug court personnel as well, to effectively deliver treatment in the community setting.

DISCUSSION QUESTIONS

1. Describe at least three critical components of the pretreatment process for drug court clients.
2. Describe the critical elements of informed consent.

3. What would best characterize the "spin" on communications between a counselor and the court regarding drug court clients?
4. How do Walker and Logan advise drug court counselors about how to approach the issue of confidentiality?

REFERENCES

Anglin, D. & Hser, Y. (1991). Criminal justice and the drug abusing offender: Policy issues of coerced treatment. *Behavioral Science Law, 9,* 243-267.

Bearhs, J.O. & Gutheil, T.G. (2001). Informed consent in psychotherapy. *American Journal of Psychiatry, 158*(2), 4-10.

Belenko, S. (1999). Research on drug courts: A critical review 1999 update. *National Drug Court Institute Review, 2*(2), 1-58.

Belenko, S. (2001). *Research on drug courts: A critical review 2001 update.* Alexandria, VA: National Drug Court Institute.

Belenko, S. (2002). Drug courts. In C.G. Leukefeld, F. Tims, & D. Farabee (Eds.), *Treatment of drug offenders* (pp. 301-318). New York: Springer Publishing.

Berg, J.W., Appelbaum, P.S., Lidz, C.W., & Parker, L.S. (2001). *Informed consent: Legal theory and clinical practice* (2nd ed.). New York: Oxford University Press.

Center on Substance Abuse Treatment. (1997). *Substance abuse treatment planning guide and checklist for treatment-based drug courts.* DHHS Publication No. SMA 97-3136. Washington, DC: U.S. Government Printing Office.

Donovan, D.M. & Rosengren, D.B. (1999). Motivation for behavior change and treatment among substance abusers. In J.A. Tucker, D.M. Donovan, & G.A. Marlatt (Eds.), *Changing addictive behavior: Bridging clinical and public health strategies* (pp. 127-159). New York: Guilford Press.

Drug Courts Program Office. (1997). *Defining drug courts: The key components.* Washington, DC: U.S. Department of Justice.

Faden, R.R. & Beauchamp, T.L. (1999). The concept of informed consent. In T.L. Beauchamp & L. Walters (Eds.), *Contemporary issues in bioethics* (5th ed.) (pp. 139-142). Belmont, CA: Wadsworth Publishing Company.

Farabee, D., Prendergast, M., & Anglin, D. (1998). The effectiveness of coerced treatment for drug-abusing offenders. *Federal Probation, 62,* 3-10.

Fishbein, D.H. (2000). *The science, treatment, and prevention of antisocial behaviors.* Kingston, NJ: Civic Research Institute.

Ginsburg, J.I.D., Mann, R.E., Rotgers, F., & Weekes, J.R. (2002). Motivational interviewing with criminal justice populations. In W.R. Miller & S. Rollnick (Eds.), *Motivational interviewing: Preparing people for change* (2nd ed.) (pp. 333-346). New York: Guilford Press.

Herman, J. (1992). *Trauma and recovery.* New York: Basic Books.

Holtzworth-Munroe, A., Smultzler, N., & Sandin, E. (1997). A brief review of the research on husband violence. *Aggression and Violent Behavior, 2*(2), 179-213.

Leshner, A. (1997). Addiction is a disease—and it matters. *Science, 278,* 45-47.

Leukefeld, C.G. & Tims, F.M. (1992). Directions for practice and research. In C.G. Leukefeld & F.M. Tims (Eds.), *Drug abuse treatment services in prisons and jails* (pp. 279-293). NIDA Monograph No. 118. Rockville, MD: National Institute on Drug Abuse.

Leukefeld, C.G., Tims, F.M., & Farabee, D. (2002). *Treatment of drug offenders: Policies and issues.* New York: Springer Publishing Co.

Leukefeld, C.G., Tims, F.M., & Platt, J.J. (2001). Future directions in substance abuse relapse and recovery. In F.M. Tims, C.G. Leukefeld, & J.J. Platt (Eds.), *Relapse and recovery in addictions* (pp. 401-413). New Haven, CT: Yale University Press.

Logan, T.K., Hoyt, W., McCollister, K., French, M., Leukefeld, C., & Minton, L. (in press). Economic evaluation of drug court: Methodology, results, and policy implications. *Evaluation and Program Planning.*

Logan, T.K., Walker, R., Cole, J., & Leukefeld, C. (2002). Victimization and substance use among women: Contributing factors, interventions, & implications. *General Review of Psychology, 6*(4), 325-397.

Logan, T., Williams, K., & Leukefeld, C. (2001). A statewide drug court needs assessment: Identifying target counties, assessing readiness. *Journal of Offender Rehabilitation, 33*(3), 1-25.

Marlowe, D.B., Glass, D.J., Merikle, E.P., Festinger, D.S., DeMatteo, D.S., Marczyk, G. R., & Platt, J.J. (2001). Efficacy of coercion in substance abuse treatment. In F.M. Tims, C.G. Leukefeld, & J.J. Platt (Eds.), *Relapse and recovery in addictions* (pp. 208-227). New Haven, CT: Yale University Press.

Miller, W.R. & Rollnick, S. (1991). *Motivational interviewing: Preparing people to change addictive behaviors.* New York: Guilford Press.

Miller, W.R. & Rollnick, S. (2002). *Motivational interviewing: Preparing people for change* (2nd ed.). New York: Guilford Press.

Polcin, D.L. (2001). Drug and alcohol offenders coerced into treatment: A review of modalities and suggestions for research on social model programs. *Substance Use and Misuse, 36,* 589-609.

Raine, A. (1994). *The psychopathology of crime.* San Diego, CA: Academic Press.

Sherin, K.M. & Mahoney, B. (1996). *Treatment drug courts: Integrating substance abuse treatment with legal case processing.* DHHS Pub. No. (SMA) 96-3113. Washington, DC: Department of Health and Human Services.

United States Department of Justice. (1997) *Defining drug courts: The key components.* Washington, DC: Department of Justice, Office of Justice Programs, Drug Courts Program Office.

van den Bree, M.B.M., Svikis, D.S., & Pickens, R. W. (2000). Antisocial personality and drug use disorders: Are they genetically related? In D.H. Fishbein (Ed.), *The science, treatment, and prevention of antisocial behaviors: Application to the criminal justice system.* Kingston, NJ: Civic Research Institute.

Walker, R. (1992a) Substance abuse and B-cluster disorders I: Understanding the dual diagnosis patient. *Journal of Psychoactive Drugs, 24*(3), 223-232.

Walker, R. (1992b). Substance abuse and B-cluster disorders II: Treatment recommendations. *Journal of Psychoactive Drugs, 24*(3), 233-241.

Walker, R. & Leukefeld, C.G. (2002). Employment rehabilitation. In C.G. Leukefeld, F.M. Tims, & D. Farabee (Eds.), *Treatment of drug offenders: Policies and issues* (pp. 69-79). New York: Springer Publishing Co.

Walker, R. & Staton, M. (2000). The concept of cultural diversity in social work ethics. *Journal on Social Work Education, 36*(3), 449-463.

Wanberg, K.W. & Milkman, H.B. (1998). *Criminal conduct and substance abuse treatment.* Thousand Oaks, CA: Sage Publications.

Yochelson, S. & Samenow, S.E. (1976). *The criminal personality* (Vol. 1). New York: Jason Aaronson.

Yochelson, S. & Samenow, S.E. (1977). *The criminal personality* (Vol. 2). New York: Jason Aaronson.

Chapter 9

Restrictive Intermediate Punishment Programming: A Community-Based Treatment Program for Substance-Addicted Correctional Clients

Barbara Sims
M. A. "Toni" DuPont-Morales

A report by the Robert Wood Johnson Foundation (2001) discusses the patterns and trends of substance abuse and reveals that abuse of drugs is the single most serious health problem in the United States. The study reports that substance abuse causes more deaths, illnesses, and disabilities than any other health problem and, unfortunately, is the least treated. Only about 25 percent of substance-addicted individuals receive treatment, although much research indicates that some treatment programs can work. Findings suggest, for example, that after six months of treatment, alcohol, cocaine, and opiate use drop by approximately 50 percent (Robert Wood Johnson Foundation, 2001). The Federal Bureau of Prisons, tracking inmates released at the end of 1995, found that only 3.3 percent of offenders who completed a residential drug abuse treatment program were likely to be rearrested in the first six months of release, compared with 12.1 percent of offenders who did not receive treatment. Further, a significant number of treated offenders (12.1 percent) were less likely to use

Funding for this research was provided by a grant from the Pennsylvania Commission on Crime and Delinquency (PCCD). Major portions of this chapter are reprinted from the final report by the authors to the PCCD with that agency's permission.

drugs in that same time period than were untreated offenders (36.7 percent) (Federal Bureau of Prisons, 1998).

Data from a 1997 survey of correctional facilities found that drug and alcohol counseling is available in 40 percent of prisons (federal, state, and local), with approximately 173,000 adults and juveniles in those programs (Office of National Drug Control Policy [ONDCP], 2001). Treatment modalities include therapeutic communities (intensive, long-term residential treatment for hard-core drug users), pharmacological maintenance programs (methadone, naltrexone, buprenorphine, etc.), outpatient treatment programs, residential treatment programs for both treatment and aftercare, and combinations of these programming types.

The underlying objective of substance abuse treatment is to release back into society addiction-free individuals who refrain from engaging in criminal activities. Important to corrections is the fact that treatment, including treatment for relapses, is far less expensive than incarceration and substance addictions that go untreated. Figures from a national study that examined the costs of such treatment, for example, suggest that at a cost of about $2,941 per treatment episode, substance abuse treatment programs result in an average savings of about three to one: every dollar spent on treatment saves society three dollars (reduced crime-related and health care costs that would have been paid for by taxpayers) (ONDCP, 2001).

According to Palmer (1996), substance abuse intervention calls for multimodality programs with increased intensity of contact by criminal justice personnel. In order for substance abuse programming to be effective, it must be realized that one size does not fit all. Treatment providers and criminal justice practitioners alike are recognizing that drug offenders are not a homogeneous group and, as such, require individualized treatment (Vigdal & Stadler, 1996). There is also an increase in the realization that substance abuse is a chronic disease and is not likely to be cured by any single program intervention. This does not mean, however, that the overly pessimistic thinking about substance abuse treatment is correct. As has been suggested here, properly implemented substance abuse programming can, in some cases, (1) reduce substance abuse in addicted offenders and (2) provide the corrections environment with an alternative to the more costly option of incarceration.

The purpose of this chapter is to describe how several Pennsylvania counties were able to implement one such substance abuse treatment program by receiving funds from the Pennsylvania Commission on Crime and Delinquency (PCCD). It outlines the process of developing a protocol for the collection of data on offenders from counties funded for pilot programs and reports preliminary findings from the first eighteen months of programming. The implications of the overall implementation process and the initial outcome data are included in the summary and conclusions section of the chapter.

REVIEW OF THE LITERATURE

From a classical theory standpoint, the criminal justice system operated, from the 1970s through the 1990s, under a deterrence model of justice. Under this model, it was thought that in order to deter crime, punishment had to be swift and certain; but more important, it had to be severe in nature. Lawmakers, both state and federal, acting under an assumption that the public would not settle for anything less than a "get tough" approach to crime in local communities, launched a war on drugs and crime that included new legislation such as mandatory minimums and three-strike laws intended to put repeat offenders behind bars for longer periods of time. It quickly became clear, as the number of correctional clients (prison, jail, or community-supervised individuals) reached a record high of 6.6 million in 2001 (Salant, 2002), that the goal of corrections would be grounded in a crime-control model of justice. Under this model, incapacitation, retribution, and both specific and general deterrence would take the place of attempts at rehabilitating individuals.

As the 1990s came to a close, the get tough approach to crime had placed a considerable burden on corrections systems across the country. The U.S. incarceration rate grew from 93 per 100,000 citizens in 1972 to about 500 per 100,000 in 2000 (Beck & Karberg, 2001). Only time, and a great deal of additional research, will tell if accelerated incarceration rates had anything to do with declining crime rates, a subject that is beyond the scope of this chapter. What is certain, however, is that higher incarceration rates produced prison systems that were overcrowded and that could provide only a minimal amount of treatment programs with "little focus on the long-term change in offenders even when some programming exists" (Palmer, 1996:8).

According to Palmer (1996), there has been a moving away from this strict crime-control/punishment model of corrections in the most recent past. He refers to this change in corrections philosophy as the "re-legitimization of intervention" and suggests that it was brought about primarily by "regained substantial scientific" inquiry (Palmer, 1996:10-11). In other words, researchers produced a body of work that pointed to one conclusion: efforts at programming can reduce recidivism in experimental (treatment) groups when compared with nontreated (control) groups. In addition, and as suggested by Palmer (1996), the rehabilitative ideal refused to die as proponents of crime-control models of justice failed to convince the public that rehabilitation should be abandoned.

Community-Based Substance Abuse Treatment Programming in the Correctional Setting

The issue of treatment for the institutional-based, substance-addicted correctional client was covered previously in earlier chapters. Many of the issues discussed in those chapters will not, then, be rehashed here. When it comes to this type of treatment, however, as may well be the case for other types of treatment programs, there is a great deal of overlap in several critical areas when it comes to delivering treatment in either the institutional or community setting.

As has been stated by several authors included in this text, effective assessment and corresponding placement in treatment that is closely matched with clients' needs is critical to producing positive outcomes for individuals with substance abuse problems. As argued by Vigdal and Stadler (1996:17-18), "The assessment must be relatively simple, reliable, valid, and fast, yet comprehensive enough to include information on several continuums." This means that any assessment tool used by corrections staff and/or treatment providers should not only identify past history of problems with substances, times in treatment, and the types of treatment programs in which the individual has been placed, but should also capture a broader profile of the offender. This profile should include, in the community corrections setting, the criminal history of the client and any history of prior probation/parole supervision. Other background information about the corrections client, including marital status, work history, and a variety of additional sociodemographic information, is needed to further assist the criminal justice community in making a determination about risks associated with clients and appropriate levels of supervision under which to place them.

It has also been noted earlier, and repeated again here because of its importance, that corrections managers must recognize that along with adequate assessment, there must be a wide variety of options available in which to place individuals because of the corresponding wide variety of presenting problems among this population. Prior to making a commitment to move toward a goal of placing substance-addicted individuals in the community for treatment, corrections managers and treatment providers alike must first assess the availability of programs in those communities.

A report by the Office of National Drug Control Policy (2002) concluded that community-based substance abuse treatment programs can work. Across eleven cities, approximately 100,000 clients were included in a study assessing outcomes of such programs. Findings indicate that, depending on treatment modality, weekly use of heroin, cocaine, and marijuana was significantly reduced. Findings also revealed a significant reduction in criminal activity (between 36 and 61 percent) and improvements in clients' employment status (between 4 and 12 percent) (ONDCP, 2002).

In a similar vein, Goldkamp, White, and Robinson (2002), through a series of focus groups with drug court clients across six sites, were able to demonstrate how this particular type of community-based treatment program can work to bring down both substance abuse and repeat offending. Several important themes emerged from this evaluation, including one important finding that these clients were individuals with very serious substance abuse problems and co-occurring problems associated with that abuse.

A second important theme is the fact that participants in the focus groups expressed a great deal of support for the drug court's approach to punishment and treatment, suggesting that the coordination between judicial supervision and treatment is an effective method of treating substance abuse (Goldkamp et al., 2002). Participants expressed more positive attitudes toward the drug court approach to treatment compared with other treatment modalities in which they had been involved, primarily because of their view that the constant threat of incarceration was a strong motivating factor in both refraining from drug use and from engaging in criminal activity while undergoing treatment (Goldkamp et al., 2002). Although self-reported estimates of number of crimes committed while in treatment varied across the six sites, overall, Goldkamp et al. (2002) concluded that only a minority of participants used drugs and committed crimes while undergoing treatment in the drug courts.

Aftercare programs for parolees have long been strongly recommended in many treatment areas, and substance abuse treatment is one of them. Whatever modicum of progress might have been made in prison or jail is sure to be short-lived if treatment does not follow the inmate into the community.

Under the Violent Crime Control and Law Enforcement Act of 1994, states were encouraged to provide treatment to correctional clients through the Residential Substance Abuse Treatment (RSAT) grants program. Findings from an early process evaluation of several such programs revealed that any gains made from prison treatment programs will be short-lived without community aftercare programs (National Institute of Justice [NIJ], 2000). The implication for community-based substance abuse treatment programming from this finding is that treatment in the community is highly recommended for individuals with histories of both substance abuse and criminal behavior.

The ONDCP (2001) documents support for such an assumption using data from the Treatment Accountability for Safer Communications (TASC) program. Just as has been found with drug courts, when treatment is combined with criminal justice supervision, it can work to prevent relapses and subsequent criminal activity. It should be noted, however, that within the TASC program, emphasis is also placed on assisting clients in finding and retaining employment and in developing and/or improving their personal and social functioning skills (ONDCP, 2001).

Within the framework of a return to the rehabilitative ideal, although caution is certainly needed before acccepting an argument that the U.S. criminal justice field has shifted from punishment as retribution to punishment as rehabilitation, treatment for correctional clients who abuse substances shows great promise. Through reliable and appropriate assessment and placement in programs that closely match offenders' needs, and through careful monitoring in the community, the corrections community can do much toward reducing both the abuse of substances and subsequent criminal behavior. In a time of crowded prisons and the host of problems that result from this overcrowding, community-based substance abuse treatment programs offer an attractive alternative to state corrections managers.

PENNSYLVANIA'S RESTRICTIVE INTERMEDIATE PUNISHMENT PROGRAM

Not unlike other states, Pennsylvania has seen an increase in its prison population. Total commitments to Pennsylvania's state prisons rose by 6 percent from 1999 to 2000, with an 8.7 percent increase in the number of inmates sentenced for twenty years or more (PA Department of Corrections, 2001a). Currently, Pennsylvania's prisons operate at approximately 142 percent of institutional capacity, with about 37,000 inmates (PA Department of Corrections, 2001a). Of the 10,486 inmates released in 2001, 70 percent had a drug and/or alcohol problem (PA Department of Corrections, 2001b).

Changes in Pennsylvania's sentencing guidelines, which became effective on August 12, 1994, included a mechanism by which the sentencing court could consider the use of a restrictive intermediate punishment as an alternative to a recommendation of incarceration. Nonviolent offenders assessed to be dependent on drugs and/or alcohol were eligible to be considered for a treatment-based restrictive intermediate punishment (RIP) in lieu of incarceration. In June 1997, under another revision of the sentencing guidelines, drug- and/or alcohol-dependent offenders sentenced at levels 3 or 4 of the guidelines became eligible to receive a sentence of RIP that includes intensive drug and alcohol treatment. Treatment is determined to be necessary through the use of an assessment in conjunction with the Pennsylvania Client Placement Criteria (PCPC). In all cases, offenders sentenced to a restrictive intermediate punishment at level 3 or 4 of the guidelines would be diverted from incarceration.

In June 1997, the PCCD announced to Pennsylvania county officials that $10 million in new state funds were available to support the development and implementation of drug and alcohol treatment-based restrictive intermediate punishment programs. In the funding announcement, the PCCD stated that these new funds would be used to support new pilot programs in a limited number of counties.

Funds available under the RIP funding announcement were to be used for the following new or expanded activities targeting levels 3 and 4 offenders:

1. drug and alcohol assessment and placement services;
2. drug and alcohol treatment services and related activities;
3. drug and alcohol testing services; and
4. criminal justice supervision services.

RIP Program Requirements

Several program requirements were established for counties receiving funds for RIP programming. First, counties had to develop a process whereby offenders are identified and targeted as potential candidates for a treatment-based RIP sentence. Second, counties were to develop procedures for conducting drug and/or alcohol assessments and clinical evaluations by qualified personnel. A minimum of three years of experience in this area was recommended by the PCCD. Third, counties were informed that they must be able to show evidence of coordination with the Single County Authority substance abuse treatment and funding systems, as well as the availability of sufficient capacity in residential and nonresidential licensed drug and alcohol treatment programs. These programs should be able to demonstrate sufficient experience in treating offenders and must ensure immediate access to treatment for those sentenced to RIP. Fourth, counties had to include a drug and/or alcohol testing component to ensure unannounced random testing of all offenders sentenced under RIP. Finally, program requirements outlined that counties demonstrate evidence of a criminal justice component that would provide for the supervision and monitoring of all RIP-sentenced offenders.

Anticipated Impact of RIP Programming

The PCCD expected that RIP programming would provide counties with postconviction alternatives to incarceration for nonviolent drug- and/or alcohol-dependent offenders who can be safely supervised in the community and that such programming could expand programs at the county level concentrating on rehabilitation of the substance-addicted offender.

THE PRESENT STUDY

In August 1997, the PCCD awarded a contract to Penn State Harrisburg, the purpose of which was to develop measures through which RIP programming could be evaluated. The authors worked closely with the PCCD staff, treatment providers, and county criminal justice personnel to develop reporting forms through which the funded counties could provide initial placement information, as well as outcome information, on all RIP clients. After a series of meetings and open discussions, it was decided that three forms would need to be developed: (1) a RIP eligibility status data reporting form; (2) a dedicated RIP form; and (3) a RIP outcome form.

Assessing RIP Client Placement:
The RIP Eligibility Status Data Reporting Form

The RIP eligibility form was used in the early stages of the RIP project in order to determine the extent to which counties were conducting assessments of clients for drug and alcohol dependency. As reported previously, and according to Vigdal and Stadler (1996), gone are the days when treatment providers merely accept all that apply for drug treatment. The current approach to assessment is multidimensional and calls for skilled staff and assessment instruments. The assessment tool must provide comprehensive information about the client along several continuums: history of drug use, prior treatment history, and prescribed method of treatment (Vigdal & Stadler, 1996).

The new RIP programs in Pennsylvania relied on the Pennsylvania Client Placement Criteria for Adults to assess the level of care and type of treatment needed for RIP clients. Experienced professionals were used to evaluate offenders and worked closely with corrections managers and staff. This collaborative effort is well documented as a critical element of successful treatment (Bureau of Justice Assistance, 1998).

Once offenders were found to be eligible for a RIP sentence, further clinical evaluations occurred to determine dependency issues.

Pennsylvania's RIP counties were asked to provide information pertaining to reasons individuals were *not* assessed for RIP treatment, as well as information about clients who were assessed for RIP treatment but not assigned to RIP. Possible reasons for nonassignment included the following:

1. not drug and/or alcohol dependent;
2. current offense or prior record;
3. detainers;
4. not approved by the judge;
5. not approved by the district attorney;
6. lack of a treatment slot;
7. the offender declined treatment; or
8. some other reason for nonassignment.

Well over a majority of assessed eligible clients were placed in RIP programming, with 3 percent listed as not being approved by a judge, 4 percent not being approved by the district attorney, 3 percent because the offender refused treatment, and 8 percent because they were assessed as not being drug or alcohol dependent. According to information reported by the RIP counties, not one offender who was assessed as being in need of treatment was refused such treatment because of the lack of a treatment slot.

Initial eligibility and assessment information is important to corrections managers. In the Pennsylvania study, the funding source had an interest in knowing if the RIP programs were following the prescribed guidelines related to assessment and placement. Further, the data collected in this early stage provided the PCCD and the treatment counties with a first look at the type of substance problems associated with RIP clients. Having this information assists corrections managers in developing a protocol for delivering community-based treatment and identifying the availability of needed treatment services found within their local areas.

Summary Information from the RIP Dedicated Form

A second form, referred to as the RIP dedicated form (DF), was developed to capture initial information about RIP clients and level of supervision. As of August 2, 2000, the Penn State Harrisburg research team had received from the participating RIP counties a total of 1,437 DFs. When examining the data file, however, it was discovered that some counties had sent duplicate information on some RIP clients. After a careful screening of the data file and deleting those clients for whom there were duplicate information, a client base of 1,208 remained.

As shown in Table 9.1, the age range of RIP clients is seventeen to sixty-six, with a mean age of thirty-two. The majority of clients are male (81 percent), with only 231 female clients (19 percent). Almost half of RIP clients are black/African American (48 percent), 24 percent are Hispanic, 28 percent are white, and less than 1 percent are reported as being from some "other" race/ethnic category. Forty-six percent of RIP clients are reported as not having a high school education, 43 percent as having finished high school, with less than 1 percent reported as being college graduates (roughly 10 percent are reported as having some college or a two-year technical degree).

TABLE 9.1. Descriptive profile of RIP offender population at program intake

Category	Percentages reported
Age	
Range = 17-66	
Mean = 32 years	
Gender	
Male	81
Female	19
Race	
White	28
Black/African American	48
Hispanic	24
Other	<1
Education	
Less than high school	46
High school graduate	43
Some college	8
Two-year degree	2
College graduate	<1

Other basic information on RIP clients not shown in Table 9.1 reveals that 89 percent moved either two or fewer times during the year prior to being sentenced to RIP, and 40 percent are reported as not having worked during that year. Only 22 percent of clients were reported as having worked eight months or longer in the year prior to sentencing. With regard to restrictive criminal justice sanctions that were added to the RIP sentence, 3 percent of clients were assigned to house arrest, 31 percent to electronic monitoring, 17 percent to both house arrest and electronic monitoring, and 32 percent had no additional restrictions added (17 percent of clients are reported as having some "other" restriction added).

In sum, the offenders who were initially placed in Pennsylvania's RIP programs were, primarily, uneducated, male, minorities in their thirties with an unstable employment and residential history. Although the criminal history of these early RIP clients is not available here, we can assume that these are not first-time offenders given the level of supervision assigned to almost two-thirds of them (described earlier as additional criminal justice sanctions added). We can also assume that the offenses committed by these clients were not of a violent nature. We can make this assumption because the PCCD guidelines called for the exclusion of violent offenders.

Prior Treatment History and Initial Level of Care

Offenders sentenced to RIP have extensive histories of prior treatment. As shown in Tables 9.2 and 9.3, 34 percent of RIP clients have

TABLE 9.2. Prior treatment history

Service received	Percent (%)
Nonintensive outpatient	34
Intensive outpatient	22
Partial hospitalization	8
Inpatient residential/halfway house	10
Inpatient hospitalized detox	18
Inpatient detox (non-hospital)	9
Medically monitored short-term residential	32
Medically monitored long-term residential	20

TABLE 9.3. Initial level of care

Service received	Percent (%)
Nonintensive outpatient	12
Intensive outpatient	17
Partial hospitalization	12
Inpatient residential/halfway house	6
Inpatient hospitalized detox	1
Inpatient detox (non-hospital)	1
Medically monitored short-term residential	24
Medically monitored long-term residential	28

been treated in a nonintensive outpatient program, with 22 percent of clients reporting having been treated through intensive outpatient means. Eight percent have been treated through "partial" hospitalization, with another 10 percent treated in inpatient hospitalization. Twenty-seven percent of RIP clients have previously undergone detox, and over half (52 percent) report having been treated in either a short- or long-term residential program.

Clearly, these clients have a long history of drug and/or alcohol abuse as well as experience in a variety of treatment programs. Given this history, it is essential to recognize the fact that there will be failures in this somewhat innovative program, no less so than what is found in other programs with similar goals (drug courts, for example).

Summary of RIP Outcome Information

A separate outcome data reporting form was developed to capture information about clients' progression through treatment. The person completing the form was asked to provide information about initial level of treatment, relapse events, including stepped-up or stepped-down supervision, and time in treatment for both *successful* and *unsuccessful* RIP clients. It should be pointed out that termination from RIP treatment was at the discretion of the supervising officer. It is probable, then, that circumstances under which clients were terminated varied greatly across the counties.

According to the outcome data file, and as of August 2000, RIP counties reported that 230 clients had successfully completed RIP programming (25 percent) and that 300 (32 percent) clients had been "unsuccessfully" terminated from RIP programming. Approximately 400 (43 percent) clients were still under RIP treatment as of August 2000 (see Table 9.4).

Table 9.5 summarizes the type of treatment in which 495 RIP clients were placed across the participating counties by whether cases were classified as either successful or unsuccessful. By far, the two most frequently used types of treatment placement for "successful" clients (205 cases) during the period reported on here, e.g., the initial stages of RIP programming in Pennsylvania, were outpatient (79; 39

TABLE 9.4. RIP outcome information

Outcome	Number	Percentage (%)
Successful	230	25
Unsuccessful	300	32
Still in treatment	400	43
Total	930	100

TABLE 9.5. Successful/unsuccessful RIP releases by initial level of care

Type of treatment	Successful cases	Unsuccessful cases
Outpatient	79	52
Intensive outpatient	100	116
Partial hospitalization	2	12
Halfway house	3	23
Medically monitored inpatient detox	0	1
Medically monitored short-term residential	5	25
Medically monitored long-term residential	15	60
Medically managed inpatient residential	1	1
Total number of cases	205	290

Note: The discrepancy between the numbers listed in this table and those listed in Table 9.4 is due to missing data on some of the cases terminated from RIP.

percent) and intensive outpatient (100; 49 percent) programs. The average length of time spent in treatment for successful RIP clients ranged from 1.8 months to 18.4 months, with an average of 8.4 months.

For unsuccessful RIP clients, and compared to the numbers reported previously, a smaller number (52; 18 percent) were placed in outpatient treatment, and slightly more cases were placed in intensive outpatient treatment (116; 40 percent). Also, there appears to be a wider range of treatment utilization than was found for the successful RIP cases, especially for medically monitored short-term residential (25; 9 percent) and medically monitored long-term residential (60; 21 percent). The average length of time in treatment, as shown in Table 9.5, for RIP failures is much shorter than was found for RIP successes. The data show that the range of time in treatment for the failures is four to ten months, with an average of 5.96 months.

These early results associated with Pennsylvania's early cohort of RIP clients are not surprising. The profile data reveal a clientele with a long history of abusing substances. A closer look at Table 9.5 suggests that of the 495 RIP clients for whom we had outcome data, over half (59 percent) required more intensive treatment and failed earlier than did their "successful" counterparts. We can conclude that relapses may occur several times before any type of progress can be seen, a finding supported by previous studies. The fact that there are some reported successes in the early stages of a new program, given the criminal and substance-abusing history of its clientele, is somewhat promising.

RIP Event History

Part of the RIP outcome reporting form asks counties for information about the history of RIP clients. The reporting form allows counties to report on step-up or step-down treatment approaches and/or levels of supervision for RIP clients. The information reported in Table 9.6 is only for outpatient, intensive outpatient, partial hospitalization, halfway house, and medically short/long-term residential initial levels of care. Recall that these are the most frequently used initial levels of care for most RIP clients.

As shown in Table 9.6, the most frequent type of first incident reported for all RIP clients is "drug use," not surprisingly followed by "failure to comply with treatment." The exception is for those clients who were placed initially in a halfway house, with only 10 percent being reported as involved with drug use in the first reported incident, or those clients who were in some sort of short/long-term residential program (only 8 percent reported to have been caught using drugs). Although there does appear to be some problem with alcohol associated with the first incident of RIP clients, clearly drug use is a much more serious problem for this group of clients.

The data in Table 9.6 also indicate that a high number of first incidents were noted as "failure to comply with treatment." The percentages are comparable in this category for outpatient-treated clients and for intensive outpatient and partial hospitalization as well. The percentages, however, are much higher for failure to comply incidents among those clients in halfway houses or in some other type of residential program. When it comes to being arrested for a new offense, and for those clients on which data were available (N = 649), note that a small percentage of clients across all treatment modalities were arrested for a felony, nondrug-related offense. Of concern, however, is the high percentages of RIP clients who were arrested, while in treatment, for a felony, drug offense coupled with felony nondrug offense.

SUMMARY AND CONCLUSIONS

We have attempted to demonstrate here how we worked with the PCCD and those counties that initially came online with RIP programming to develop a means through which to report information on (1) how eligibility of RIP clients is determined; (2) number of clients by county placed in RIP programming; (3) initial level of care for RIP clients; (4) success/failure rate of RIP clients; (5) length of time in treatment for RIP clients; and (6) first-incident histories of RIP clients. Returning to the stated goals by the PCCD for RIP programs, we can conclude from the preliminary data that the counties are assessing offenders for drug and/or alcohol dependency following PCPC guidelines for assessment and that no eligible offenders are being denied a RIP sentence due to lack of a treatment slot. We can further conclude that close supervision of RIP clients has been undertaken in

TABLE 9.6. RIP event history by level of care—First incident

Level of care	Type of incident	Number	Percent (%)
Outpatient	Drug use	48	37
	Alcohol use	4	3
	Failure to comply with treatment	30	23
	Misdemeanor arrest	4	3
	Felony drug/nondrug arrest	41	32
Intensive outpatient	Drug use	94	41
	Alcohol use	2	<1
	Failure to comply with treatment	60	26
	Misdemeanor arrest	6	3
	Felony drug arrest	3	1
	Felony nondrug arrest	4	2
	Felony drug/nondrug arrest	57	25
Partial hospitalization	Drug use	23	52
	Alcohol use	5	11
	Failure to comply with treatment	12	27
	Misdemeanor arrest	2	4
	Felony drug arrest	1	2
	Felony nondrug arrest	1	2
Halfway house	Drug use	4	10
	Alcohol use	4	10
	Failure to comply with treatment	21	53
	Misdemeanor arrest	1	2
	Felony drug arrest	1	2
	Felony nondrug arrest	1	2
	Felony drug/nondrug arrest	8	20

TABLE 9.6 *(continued)*

Level of care	Type of incident	Number	Percent (%)
Medically monitored short/long-term residential	Drug use	17	8
	Alcohol use	2	<1
	Failure to comply with treatment	97	46
	Misdemeanor arrest	—	—
	Felony drug arrest	8	4
	Felony nondrug arrest	1	<1
	Felony drug/nondrug arrest	87	41

the field, with an adequate reporting of step-up and/or step-down treatment modalities along with criminal justice supervision services. Thus these pilot Pennsylvania RIP programs appear to be meeting the overall goals of implementing this type of programming.

Although the outcome data we initially gathered on behalf of the PCCD should be viewed with much caution because it is indeed preliminary in nature and thus should not be seen as part of an evaluation of RIP programming, we can conclude that RIP programs are meeting, at least in part, another important goal. These programs are providing corrections managers an alternative to incarceration for nonviolent substance-addicted offenders.

There is, however, a cautionary tale here. These early data suggest that RIP clients are individuals who have long been struggling with problems associated with both addiction and criminal behavior. The rearrest figures are quite disturbing, not to mention the relapse data. Clearly, for some offenders, RIP programming does not appear to work well. We suggest that the current and subsequent data be examined more closely, in particular when it comes to the past criminal history. It could very well be that, upon closer inspection, some RIP clients should receive treatment within a more secure environment, reserving community treatment slots for those individuals with a more stable background.

The good news is that RIP programming is working for many community correctional clients. A weeding out of the higher-risk offenders could, quite possibly, serve these counties well and not put at risk the loss of critical support and resources for this attractive alternative to incarceration. Given the increase in prison capacity in Pennsylvania, and other states as well, diverting low-risk offenders to a community-based alternative seems reasonable. Sufficient research-based information now points to a conclusion that these alternatives can work as long as they are implemented correctly and meet the many needs of the substance-addicted indivdiual.

DISCUSSION QUESTIONS

1. Sims and DuPont-Morales appear to be arguing for an expansion of community-based substance abuse treatment programs. What, do they suggest, is the major argument for such programming?
2. Describe the basic criteria for funding to Pennsylvania counties wishing to implement restrictive intermediate punishment (RIP) programs.
3. From the data presented by the authors, how would you describe the successful RIP client?
4. In their summary and conclusions, Sims and DuPont-Morales state, "These pilot Pennsylvania RIP programs appear to be meeting the overall goal of providing counties with an alternative to incarceration for nonviolent substance-addicted offenders." Using the data presented in this chapter, argue for or against the authors' general conclusion.

REFERENCES

Beck, A. & Karberg, J. (2001). *Bureau of Justice Statistics bulletin: Prison and jail inmates at midyear 2000.* Washington, DC: U.S. Department of Justice.

Bureau of Justice Assistance. (1998). *Critical elements in the planning, development, and implementation of successful correctional options.* Washington, DC: U.S. Department of Justice.

Federal Bureau of Prisons. (1998). *TRIAD drug treatment evaluation six-month report: Executive summary.* Washington, DC: U.S. Department of Justice.

Goldkamp, J.S., White, M.D., & Robinson, J.B. (2002). *An honest chance: Perspectives on drug courts.* Washington, DC: Bureau of Justice Statistics. Available at <bja.ncjrs.org/publications>.

National Institute of Justice. (2000, July). Reducing offender drug use through prison-based treatment. *NIJ Journal,* pp. 21-22.

Office of National Drug Control Policy. (2001). *Drug treatment in the criminal justice system.* Washington, DC: Executive Office of the President.

Office of National Drug Control Policy. (2002). *National drug control strategy.* Washington, DC: Executive Office of the President.

Palmer, T. (1996). Growth-centered intervention: An overview of changes in recent decades. In K.E. Early (Ed.), *Drug treatment behind bars: Prison-based strategies for change* (pp. 7-16). Westport, CT: Praeger.

Pennsylvania Department of Corrections. (2001a). *Annual statistics.* Camp Hill, PA: Author.

Pennsylvania Department of Corrections. (2001b). *Portrait of an inmate returning to the community.* Camp Hill, PA: Author.

Robert Wood Johnson Foundation. (2001). *Substance abuse: The nation's number one health problem.* Princeton, NJ: Author.

Salant, J. (2002, August 25). More Americans on parole in jail by the end of 2001. *Austin American Statesman,* p. A5.

Vigdal, G.L. & Stadler, D.W. (1996). Assessment, client treatment matching, and managing the substance abusing offender. In K.E. Early (Ed.), *Drug treatment behind bars: Prison-based strategies for change* (pp. 17-43). Westport, CT: Praeger.

PART IV:
SPECIAL TREATMENT POPULATIONS

This fourth and final part of this text deals with treating both the juvenile and the female substance-addicted correctional client. As has been pointed out in many of the preceding chapters, it is clear that if treatment is going to work, it must be better tailored to meet the needs of individual clients. It has been shown that what might work for adult males probably will not work for young, adolescent males. Nor do adult- and male-based treatment programs meet the needs of females, more especially those of the adolescent female. It does appear that the field of corrections is beginning to accept the fact that more needs to be done in the area of needs assessment, and this is especially true for these heretofore grossly underrepresented groups. With careful assessment, coupled with individualized treatment needs, substance abuse programming can, just as any other treatment program, work to produce a positive outcome for younger correctional clients and for female substance abusers as well.

In Chapter 10, Glaser and Cohen present a model for treating juvenile substance abuse in the institutional setting. They list the major components of a program that have been pulled from the literature on the subject and suggest a comprehensive approach that begins with careful screening and pretraining and moves toward a careful implementation of a multiprone group content curriculum. The authors contend that because this particular program is grounded in the best practices identified in the field that it is a step in the right direction for treatment of juveniles who abuse substances.

In Chapter 11, Calhoun, Stefurak, and Johnson focus on treating the adolescent female. As suggested by the authors, the Gaining Insight into Relationships for Lifelong Success (GIRLS) program addresses the internal needs of clients such as depression, and it pays particular attention to gender-specific presenting problems. Baletka and Shearer, in Chapter 12, focus on the adult female substance-addicted institutional client. They point out that most prisons are ill equipped to treat females and that they miss the mark when trying to simply implement programs designed for male inmates. Through careful design, testing, and evaluating of the Female Offender Critical Intervention Inventory (FOCI), Baletka and Shearer demonstrate the importance of needs assessment for the female inmate who has been found to be addicted to drugs and/or alcohol.

Chapter 10

Treating Juvenile Substance Abuse in the Institutional Setting

Brian A. Glaser
Paul J. Cohen

According to recent epidemiological statistics, one-half of all high school students report using alcohol within the past thirty days, and one-quarter report using marijuana (MacKay, Fingerhut, & Duran, 2000). It should not be surprising that of an estimated 2.5 million arrests of persons under the age of eighteen in 1999, 408,800 juveniles were arrested for alcohol- and drug-related charges (Office of Juvenile Justice and Delinquency Prevention [OJJDP], 2000). This statistic does not include the vast number of juveniles who were arrested on other charges when drugs and alcohol were involved. Short-term correctional facilities are faced with the frontline problem of addressing the health and treatment of these youth. How can providers prevent adolescents who are detained on such charges from repeated involvement with illegal substances? This chapter describes an alcohol and drug group treatment program that has been developed for adolescents in a short-term, all-male regional youth detention center.

REVIEW OF THE LITERATURE

Research has suggested that several factors are associated with adolescent substance abuse. Margolis (1995) found that family dysfunction plays a crucial role in chemical dependence, especially with adolescents. Frequently more than one substance abuser is present in the home. In addition, family members become locked in dysfunctional roles. Sanjuan and Langenbucher (1999) discuss how the distinction between use and abuse is particularly important with adolescents. It has been found that youthful experimentation is common. Most juveniles use psychoactive substances and do not develop significant problems. However, the earlier the age of onset of use, the greater the likelihood that substance use may turn into abuse.

Recently, Glaser, Calhoun, and Petrocelli (2002) closely examined scale scores of the Minnesota Multiphasic Personality Inventory–Adolescent (Butcher et al., 1992) in order to isolate the personality differences that differentiate male juvenile offenders with respect to their adjudicated offense type: drug, person, or property. That is, how are offenders with substance abuse issues different from other offenders? Results of both univariate and discriminant analyses suggested that male juvenile offenders who have high degrees of psychomotor retardation (feeling immobilized and withdrawn, lacking energy to cope, and lacking hostile or aggressive impulses), and serious adolescent-school problems (poor grades, suspensions, truancy, negative attitudes toward teachers, dislike of school), are more likely to engage in drug offenses than in property crimes or crimes against other people.

Glaser et al. (2002) also found that a greater interest in manipulative and self-oriented behavior (amorality) and a greater proneness for developing alcohol and drug problems (alcohol/drug problem proneness) were more strongly associated with male juvenile offenders who were adjudicated with drug-related crimes and crimes against people in comparison to juvenile offenders adjudicated with property offenses. Higher scores on the Somatic Complaints scale also combined with psychomotor retardation and adolescent-school problem dimensions to maximally differentiate juvenile offenders adjudicated with drug offenses from juvenile offenders adjudicated with crimes against people. Such personality variables, which appear to differentiate between juvenile offenders adjudicated with drug offenses and those adjudicated with property or person offenses, are important to consider in reaching a deeper understanding of male juvenile offenders with drug-related offenses.

The goal of prevention or treatment efforts is to decrease the number of risk factors while increasing the protective factors (Sanjuan & Langenbucher, 1999). Though risk and protective factors can exert their effects in a variety of ways that are not completely understood at this time, some general characteristics have been consistently identified across studies (Padina, 1996). Risk and protective factors vary across cultural and socioeconomic groups, as well as geographic location of the offender. Greater pretreatment severity of drug use, criminal history, early onset of use, educational failure, low perception of family independence, and high perception of family control are all risk factors and have been shown to predict poor treatment outcome. Factors operating during treatment that predict better outcome (protective factors) include motivation, perceived choice in seeking treatment, rapport with clinician or staff, special services (education, vocational training, relaxation training, recreation), and parental involvement (Catalano, Hawkins, Wells, Miller, & Brewer, 1991).

Problems Associated with Treatment in Secure Juvenile Detention Centers

Due to several dramatic changes in mental health delivery systems, brief therapeutic treatment has become a necessity. Whether it is the search for a quick fix to solve a problem or a third party limiting the amount of time spent in therapy, brief or short-term therapy is no longer a trend but rather a fixture. Economic and social pressures demand that whatever is wrong be "fixed" as quickly and as cost-effectively as possible. In addressing addiction and addictive behaviors in particular, Bien, Miller, and Tonigan (1993) found that brief interventions could be effective for substance users. Grayson (1993) described short-term group counseling as a process in which each session may be independent of previous or subsequent sessions, and a participant need not go through a whole series of sessions to benefit. This principle means that each session must be well planned and carried out to ensure maximum effectiveness. Consistent with this self-contained principle, McMurran and Hollin (1993) described a modular approach in which clients may enter and leave the modular sequence at any point, thus allowing clients to be matched with appropriate components of intervention. This structure of treatment is particularly useful in settings such as short-term detention centers where the average stay for an adolescent is approximately one month before he or she moves on to another placement in the juvenile justice system.

According to Lester and Van Voorhis (1992), the benefits of group therapy with offenders are twofold: economic and therapeutic. That is, treating offenders in groups is cheaper than individual therapy, and group counseling exposes the offender to therapeutic feedback from the group. Lipsey (1992) found that juvenile delinquency treatment programs that hold more frequent sessions and are longer in duration are associated with better outcomes. In some ways, brief therapy for substance abuse is an oxymoron. That is, youths do not get to where they are in a brief period of time, so it does not seem reasonable that effective treatment can be brief. However, when it comes to treating youth in short-term facilities, providers are forced to choose between short-term therapeutic treatment and no therapeutic intervention at all.

There are limitations associated with group counseling interventions in general and with the juvenile offender population specifically. Group counseling as an intervention poses several risks. Unlike individual counseling, confidentiality cannot be ensured in a group setting; in fact, others can misuse information disclosed by a member of a group of juvenile offenders. Strong leadership can prevent such problems and protect members from coercion. Another area of concern is the volatility of adolescents in a group setting. As a result, security measures must be in place because, as in any setting with adolescents, tempers can flare. A final area of concern is the potential iatrogenic effect of grouping high-risk adolescents together (Dishion, McCord, & Poulin, 1999). That is, leaders must ensure that the groups are not used for "deviancy training."

McMurran (1991) noted that a didactic, classroom-based education does not suit adolescent offenders well. Many of the youth have learning problems and attention problems. Juvenile offenders typically do not perform well in academic settings. Groups that are structured in a classroom format may not be optimally effective or beneficial for these youth. Effective interventions are active, interactive, and skills based. If at all possible, interventions should be conducted in more natural environments than classrooms with rows of desks.

According to Hollin and Howells (1996), most successful studies of groups, while behavioral in orientation, include a cognitive component to focus on countering attitudes, values, and beliefs that support and maintain delinquent behaviors. Behavioral interventions such as relapse prevention, skills training, and anger-control training have shown to be promising, as are elements of family therapy, educational and vocational rehabilitation, and medications for coexisting psychiatric disorders. Andrews et al. (1990) suggest that nondirective client-centered therapies are to be avoided within general samples of offenders. Most groups that involve offenders need some sort of structure in which the group leaders can invoke organization and keep content moving toward certain set goals. Roberts and Camasso (1991) noted that effective programs also include an element of family work. Unfortunately, with incarcerated youth, it is often difficult to get family involvement because the legal problems are often blamed on the incarcerated youth and family members do not feel that it is their responsibility to be a part of any rehabilitation.

Given the current nature of the corrections environment, and in particular that of the juvenile delinquent, there is a need for the development of substance abuse treatment programs with potential for long-term positive outcomes though delivered in the short term. Our goal in developing such a program was to incorporate elements of what has been proven to work with the treatment of youth in the community and to adapt them to fit into a short-term detention center setting. Our model, the Juvenile Counseling and Assessment Program, is described here.

A DESCRIPTION OF THE JUVENILE COUNSELING AND ASSESSMENT PROGRAM (JCAP): A SHORT-TERM TREATMENT PROGRAM FOR SUBSTANCE-ABUSING YOUTH

The JCAP model of providing counseling services to juvenile offenders is a holistic approach (Calhoun, Glaser, & Bartolomucci, 2001). At a short-term juvenile detention center, we implemented a group counseling approach to address substance abuse with incarcerated youth, and in doing so, we have incorporated elements from those treatment approaches that have been shown to be effective.

Screening and Pretraining

The first step in creating a group involves deciding how many members will make up the group. Once the number of members in a counseling group exceeds seven or eight, any attempt by the group counselor to structure or intervene during a group session becomes increasingly difficult to initiate or to bring to fruition (Gazda, Ginter, & Horne, 2001). Maintaining therapeutic control is crucial when dealing with incarcerated youth who tend to perpetuate and amplify one another's actions, good or bad. These therapeutic challenges are further compounded by the high rates of attention-deficit/hyperactivity disorder, educational problems, and behavior disorders often exhibited in detained adolescents.

We recommend, then, eight youth as the optimal membership with two group counselors at each group session. There is always the potential for group volatility. Lower numbers make the group safer, as well as keeping the group process flowing toward the set goals of the group.

Before the group can commence, each member must be screened. Not all juvenile offenders are suitable for group-based treatment (Hollin, 1990). Including all possible adolescents with no selection criteria will inflate the failure rate. Our approach to screening involves a weekly mental health treatment team meeting in which we discuss, in addition to individual youths' mental health issues, the appropriateness of individuals for group membership. Any information about the youth, including data gleaned from the intake interview and clinical observations of the staff, are crucial in determining which youth are appropriate for referral to the substance abuse group. Supplemental information can also be useful. As part of each youth's intake to the facility, he is administered the Behavioral Assessment Scale for Children (BASC) (Reynolds & Kamphaus, 1992) and the University of Rhode Island Change Assessment (URICA) (McConnaughy, DiClemente, Prochaska, & Velicer, 1989). The BASC is a 186-item self-report questionnaire for adolescents designed to facilitate the differential diagnosis and classification of a variety of emotional and behavioral disorders in children and to aid in the formulation of treatment plans. The URICA is a questionnaire that evaluates the youth's readiness for change and identifies the stage the individual is at within the continuum of the change process. Both instruments are useful in determining who is appropriate for group and, perhaps more important, who is not appropriate for group.

Once the group members have been selected for appropriateness, the first meeting held is devoted to pretraining. Pretraining involves discussing group norms and basic skills and rules needed to effectively participate in a group. We have found, as have others (Gazda et al., 2001), that time invested in pretraining increases overall efficiency of the group.

Goal Setting and Building Cohesion

Goal setting and building cohesion are important parts of the group counseling process. Despite the fact that goal setting and cohesion building are an evolutionary process that occurs throughout the group, it is important to address these topics early on so that the group members maintain awareness and focus. Typically, goals for youth imposed by society and law are not the same as the goals that the youth want for themselves. Though complete cessation of all substance activity might be the desired end result of society (and of the group leaders), better decision making may eventually lead the youth to healthier decisions in the future and may serve as more realistic goals for short-term group treatment. For example, Hollin and Henderson (1984) found that it is possible to produce good outcomes in terms of improved psychological adjustment or social skills yet still have little or no effect on recidivism or further delinquency.

It is our opinion that a didactic, lecture type of interaction with the youth will not be effective. It is also believed that education about drugs and alcohol is necessary information to learn, but that information by itself is not sufficient to deter a youth from using in the future. It is also necessary to discuss each youth's personal situation that elicits drug/alcohol abuse. Many juvenile offenders who are involved with drugs and/or alcohol have several risk factors that must be addressed, and though many have limited protective factors, optimal use of any protective factors that are present should also be explored.

Roles of Group Leaders

It is important for group members to view the relationship with the group leaders not as one of authority figures preaching right and wrong but as an egalitarian relationship in which the leaders facilitate growth and change. This is very difficult in an institutional setting. However, with our groups, the leaders have a good working relationship with staff at the detention center, yet we are not perceived as staff or authority figures by the youth. It is believed that this is a key factor

in facilitating a solid working relationship with the youth. When appropriate, allowing the youth to step to the forefront and lead the
group is important.

Numerous publications have cited the effectiveness of peer-led
groups with adolescents. Redl (1945) found that therapeutic group
techniques with delinquents are beneficial because many adolescents
have been found to be more readily influenced by their peers than by
adults. Offenders who have committed similar crimes can often break
through this denial and resistance where professional counselors fail.
The proven effectiveness of peer-led groups is why, if at all possible,
it is important to encourage peers to step up in the group and discuss
the "story" of the process that they have been through with their own
struggles with substance use.

Many students begin their participation in the alcohol and drug
groups by glorifying their history of drug use. Group leaders often do
not have to address glorification because group members who have
previously attended the group generally address such bravado directly. On the other hand, the same youth who initially glorify drug
use also often display an initial defensiveness about drug use. It is the
group leaders' job to help youths feel like they are not being judged
by their past actions. The more the group leader maintains control of
the group, the more likely an atmosphere in which the group members will take risks in their disclosure will be facilitated (Gazda et al.,
2001).

As Gazda et al. (2001) noted, the most important stance that the
group counselor can take is one in which he or she does not view
himself or herself as the ultimate catalyst to resulting change in the
group members. It is of utmost importance to allow the group dynamics to evolve in such a way that the group is responsible for creating
an atmosphere that is conducive to change. The group leaders are
there to guide this process and to make certain that the process stays
on track toward the desired change.

Termination and New Member Transition

Because these groups take place at a temporary detention facility,
group members frequently leave prematurely and new members join
each session. As a result, it is necessary to treat each group as if it will
be the last time each individual member will attend. Each group ses-

sion is interconnected to previous sessions, but it is not necessary to attend previous sessions to benefit from subsequent sessions. That is, the modules are specifically designed to be delivered to an open group (one in which membership varies from session to session), as opposed to a closed group (one in which the membership does not vary across sessions). As one group member leaves, it is important to discuss with the youth how this affects the dynamics of the group. Before any new member joins the group, it is the group leaders' responsibility to allow the new member to go through the same pretraining that all members have gone through.

When a new member joins the group, however, it becomes the group's responsibility to describe group norms and what is expected from him related to those norms. It is this peer-led instruction that new members are most likely to follow. When new members view how the others are invested in the group and become comfortable with the process, it becomes easier for the new members to become engaged. As new members exhibit behavior consistent with the early stages of joining the group (glorification of substance use, defensiveness, etc.), seasoned members are able to effectively assist in confronting and facilitating progress under the guidance and supervision of the leaders.

Group Content Curriculum in the JCAP

Group content centers around five themes: (1) family issues; (2) context (triggers) of the drug/alcohol abuse; (3) conflict resolution and anger management; (4) life skills, including effective communication and social skills (Dishion, Reid, & Patterson, 1988), and (5) building strength and resiliency/future directions. Each of these themes constitutes a topic for the five-module cycle of groups as demonstrated in Table 10.1 along with the major characteristics for those themes. These areas are meant to provide a comprehensive framework for resolving the issues that contribute to the youth's pursuit of substance use.

As shown in Table 10.1, module 1 is meant to deal specifically with the home environment of the youth. Questions about how parents view the use of drugs and how the youth is disciplined when drug use is discovered are important issues to be brought out into the open and dealt with in a comfortable and trusting setting. In modules 2 and

TABLE 10.1. Outline of the content for the proposed Juvenile Counseling and Assessment Program for short-term detention facilities

Modules	Course content
1. Family issues	Parental attitudes toward drugs (neglect, disapproval, enabling)
	Parental monitoring
	Other substance abusers in home
	Conflict in the home
2. Context (triggers) of the drug/alcohol abuse	Peer usage of drugs/alcohol
	Perceived reasons for substance abuse, e.g., partying, self-medicating
	Locations and cues for using including identifying emotional states associated with using
	Marketing and financial aspects
	Level of motivation for change
	Issues of grief and loss (consequences of involvement with substance abuse, destruction of relationships)
3. Conflict resolution and anger management	Faith and personal values in conflict with substance use
	Impaired judgment
	Heightened emotionality/impulsivity
4. Life skills, including effective communication and social skills	Assertiveness training including inoculation role-playing
	Decision making
	Strained interpersonal relationships
	Interference with daily functioning in school and work performance
	Physical health, including cognitive impairment and athletic participation

Modules	Course content
5. Building strength and resiliency/future directions	Coping with life change after the cessation of use (family and peer expectations)
	Establishing protective factors
	Development of an individualized sobriety plan with probation officer for bridge from detention to community
	Dealing with community expectations/labeling
	Taking responsibility for dealing with legal consequences

3, youths are encouraged to think about how best to deal with "triggers" that bring about substance use and how to resolve conflict without resorting to anger and/or violent behavior, respectively.

A great deal of attention is given to the development of adequate social and coping skills in module 4. As indicated in Table 10.1, youth are introduced to not only assertiveness training but also a closer look at the decision-making process and how certain decisions can negatively impair daily functioning and physical health. Communication skills are stressed as an avenue toward repairing broken or strained relationships with family or friends.

SUMMARY AND CONCLUSIONS

We argue here that it is important to give detained juvenile offenders with substance abuse issues an effective counseling experience during this brief window of *imposed sobriety*. Skilled leadership is needed to (1) maintain therapeutic control; (2) prevent breaches of confidentiality; and (3) prevent iatrogenic effects (deviancy training). Each group session ends with a message of how to pursue sobriety. The main goal of the group course content is to encourage youths to take advantage of protective factors within themselves, their families, their schools, and ultimately their communities in order to maintain the sobriety imposed by detention once they leave the short-term detention facility.

Farrington and Hawkins (1991) have found that conventional involvement in family, school, church, work, and with other nonoffending peers can facilitate growth out of problematic levels of delinquent behavior. In the JCAP program, efforts are made to bridge the transition from detention to the community in several ways, not the least of which, as shown in Table 10.1 (module 5), is by assisting the youth to create a sobriety plan to be followed closely in the outside world. Furthermore, youths should engage in an in-depth exploration of how they might face unexpected reactions from their family and peers in light of their decision not to use drugs and/or alcohol. It could very well be that the youth's family members and friends are, after all, still using alcohol and/or drugs and may not be prepared to change their own behavior when in the presence of the youth. This message needs to be shared with the youth and a plan developed to assist him with dealing with any negative consequences associated with others' reactions to his sobriety.

It should be noted that we are not advocating for the quick fix method of treatment for young people who abuse substances. Yet it does appear that many incarcerated youth are presenting problems associated with substance abuse, and the fact that most nonviolent youth are imprisoned for short periods of time seems to call for an approach to treatment that can be folded into this particular scenario. Although there has been no formal evaluation of the program we have developed and that is currently being followed in at least one secure juvenile detention center, it does show promise. The fact that much of the group course curriculum has been developed by relying on identified best practices in the wider substance abuse literature puts it, at the very least, on a solid foundation. We believe, then, that the JCAP is a step in the right direction.

DISCUSSION QUESTIONS

1. Describe some of the problems associated with substance abuse treatment for juveniles held in secure detention centers.
2. According to Glaser and Cohen, what is the importance of the group leader in the short-term treatment program they describe here?
3. How does the JCAP program attempt to ease the youth's transition from detention back into the community?

REFERENCES

Andrews, D.A., Zinger, I., Hoge, R.D., Bonta, J., Gendreau, P., & Cullen, F.T. (1990). Does correctional treatment work? A clinically relevant and psychologically informed meta-analysis. *Criminology, 28,* 369-404.

Bien, T. H., Miller, W.R., & Tonnigan, J.S. (1993). Brief interventions for alcohol problems: A review. *Addiction, 88,* 315-36.

Butcher, J.N., Williams, C.L., Graham, J.R., Archer, R., Tellegen, A., Ben-Porath, Y., & Kaemmer, B. (1992). *Minnesota Multiphasic Personality Inventory—Adolescent—MMPI-A: Manual for administration, scoring and interpretation.* Minneapolis: University of Minnesota Press.

Calhoun, G.B., Glaser, B.A., & Bartolomucci, C.L. (2001). The Juvenile Counseling and Assessment Program: Collaborative treatment for juvenile offenders. *Journal of Counseling and Development, 79,* 131-141.

Catalano, R.F., Hawkins, J.D., Wells, E.A., Miller, J., & Brewer, D. (1991). Evaluation of the effectiveness of adolescent drug abuse treatment, assessment of risks for relapse, and promising approaches for relapse prevention. *International Journal of Addictions, 25*(9a&10a), 1085-1140.

Dishion, T., McCord, J., & Poulin, F. (1999). When interventions harm: Peer groups and problem behavior. *American Psychologist, 54*(9), 755-764.

Dishion, T., Reid, J.B., & Patterson, G.R. (1988). Empirical guidelines for a family intervention for adolescent drug use. *Journal of Chemical Dependency Treatment, 1*(2), 189-224.

Farrington, D.P. & Hawkins, J.D. (1991) Predicting participation, early onset, and later persistence in officially recorded offending. *Criminal Behaviour and Mental Health, 1*(1), 1-33.

Gazda, G.M., Ginter, E.J., & Horne, A.M. (2001). *Group counseling and group psychotherapy.* Boston: Allyn & Bacon.

Glaser, B.A., Calhoun, G.B., & Petrocelli, J.V. (2002). On the identification of adjudicated offenses of delinquent boys with the MMPI-A. *Criminal Justice and Behavior, 29*(2), 183-201.

Grayson, E.S. (1993). *Short term group counseling.* Laurel, MD: American Counseling Association.

Hollin, C. (1990). *Cognitive behavioral interventions with young offenders.* New York: Pergamon Press.

Hollin, C.R. & Henderson, M. (1984). Social skills training with young offenders: False expectations and the "failure of treatment." *Behavioural Psychotherapy, 12,* 331-341.

Hollin, C.R. & Howells, K. (1996). Young offenders: A clinical approach. In C. Hollin & K. Howells (Eds.), *Clinical approaches to working with young offenders* (pp. 1-5). New York: John Wiley and Sons.

Lester, D. & Van Voorhis, P. (1992). Group and milieu therapy. In D. Lester, M. Braswell, & P. Van Voorhis (Eds.), *Correctional counseling* (pp. 175-193). Cincinnati, OH: Anderson Publishing.

Lipsey, M.W. (1992). The effect of treatment on juvenile delinquents: Results from meta-analysis. In F. Loesel & D. Bender (Eds.), *Psychology and law: International perspectives* (pp. 131-143). Berlin: Walter de Gruyter.

MacKay, A.P., Fingerhut, L.A., & Duran, L.A. (2000). *Adolescent health chartbook, health, United States, 2000.* Hyattsville, MD: National Center for Health Statistics 2000.

Margolis, R. (1995). Adolescent chemical dependence: Assessment, treatment, and management. *Psychotherapy: Theory, Research, Practice, and Training, 32,* 172-179.

McConnaughy, E.A., DiClemente, C.C., Prochaska, J.O., & Velicer, W.F. (1989). Stages of change in psychotherapy: A follow-up report. *Psychotherapy, 26,* 494-503.

McMurran, M. (1991). Young offenders and alcohol-related crime: What interventions will address the issues? *Journal of Adolescence, 14,* 245-253.

McMurran, M. & Hollin, C.R. (1993). *Young offenders and alcohol: A practitioner's guidebook.* Chichester, UK: Wiley.

Office of Juvenile Justice and Delinquency Prevention 2001, Juvenile Justice Bulletin. (2000, April). Prevention of serious and violent juvenile offending. Retrieved October 19, 2000, from <http://www.ncjrs.org/html/ojjdp/jjbul2000_04_1/pag3.html>.

Padina, R.J. (1996, September). Risk and protective factor models in adolescent drug use: Putting them to work for prevention. Paper presented at the National Conference on Drug Abuse Prevention Research, Washington, DC.

Redl, F. (1945). The psychology of gang formation and the treatment of juvenile delinquents. *Psychoanalytic Study of the Child, 1,* 367-377.

Reynolds, C.R. & Kamphaus, R.W. (1992). *Behavior assessment system for children* [Instrument]. Circle Pines, MN: American Guidance Service, Inc.

Roberts, A.R. & Camasso, M.J. (1991). The effect of juvenile offender treatment programs on recidivism: A meta-analysis of 46 studies. *Notre Dame Journal of Law, Ethics and Public Policy, 5,* 421-441.

Sanjuan, P.M. & Langenbucher, J.W. (1999). Age-limited populations: Youth, adolescents, and older adults. In B.S. McCrady & E.E. Epstein (Eds.), *Addictions: A comprehensive guidebook* (pp. 477-498). New York: Oxford University Press.

Chapter 11

The Effectiveness of Substance Abuse Counseling for the Adolescent Female

Georgia Calhoun
Tres Stefurak
Cheryl Deluca Johnson

Adolescent female offenders have largely been ignored throughout the juvenile justice field. An understanding of the essential role of relationships in the development of female adolescents is needed in order to understand the role of problem behaviors in their lives (Brown & Gilligan, 1992). Without this understanding, girls are often misunderstood and mistreated, while their true needs go unnoticed. Understanding the relational context in which female juvenile offenders function may aid in the conceptualization of the challenges they have experienced in their most important relationships, providing critical treatment implications. The purpose of this chapter is to describe the use of a relational group therapy model as a means of addressing issues of drug and alcohol use with female juvenile offenders. Supporting data and a description of treatment modules are provided.

Juvenile offending by females increased during the 1990s at a rate four times that of male juvenile offenders (Stone, 1998). In 1995, female juvenile offenders represented 26 percent of all juvenile offenses. Although status offenses (those offenses that if committed by an adult would not be a crime, e.g., truancy from school, running away from home) remain the predominant charge for this population, there has been a dramatic increase of female participation in violent offenses (Bartolomucci, 2002).

The vast majority of research in the field of juvenile justice has not conceptualized female delinquency independently from male delinquency (Chesney-Lind & Sheldon, 1998). Programming and treatment for female juvenile offenders that emanated from such research were based largely on male samples and the results generalized to any females that happened to need intervention. The outcome of this practice was a masculine conceptualization of the etiology of female juvenile offending (Chesney-Lind & Sheldon, 1998).

In addition to the masculine conceptualization so often utilized with juvenile offenders, the focus has primarily been on the behaviors exhibited by the juveniles rather than the emotions fueling these behaviors. When family, school, and peer relations are discussed in male delinquency, the focus is on the problematic behavior in each realm rather than the problematic relationships that contribute to this behavior. Therefore, the intervention typically focuses on reducing these external problems through specific treatment, e.g., anger management (Calhoun, Glaser, & Bartolomucci, 1999). Such treatments, while effective in addressing these particular behaviors, do not address underlying relationship issues or emotional concerns.

DRUG AND ALCOHOL ISSUES

Alcoholism and drug addiction have long been recognized as major social problems, and the research on this subject is enormous. However, most of this research has been conducted on males (McDonough & Russell, 1994; Swift, Copeland, & Hall, 1996) and most of the treatment models were researched and developed by men (Kauffman, Silver, & Poulin, 1997; Swift et al., 1996). When women have been studied, they have been treated as a special population and are studied as a deviant from the norm of white males in addiction literature (Bushway & Heiland, 1995). Even Alcoholics Anonymous (AA), one of the most widely recognized treatment programs, reflects male attitudes about alcoholism. For example, AA focuses on powerlessness, self-sacrifice, and dependency (Kauffman et al., 1997), which may be in opposition to what women and adolescent females in recovery need, even though 40 percent of its members under the age of thirty are female (Blume, 1998).

Where gender differences have been examined among alcohol abusers, it has been found that males and females drink for different reasons (Corbin, McNair, & Carter, 1996; Beckman, 1994a). This is possibly due in part to a difference in alcohol expectancies, the anticipated outcomes of alcohol consumption. Thombs (1993) found that the strongest expectancy among females was arousal and power, while the strongest expectancy among males was physical and social pleasure. Females who were classified as problem drinkers were strongly motivated by expectancies that included feeling better about themselves, reducing stress, and increasing sociability. Their male counterparts were motivated by expectancies that included only stress reduction and increased sociability.

Given these gender differences in reasons for drinking, what might be the cause of female problem drinkers seeking to feel better about themselves and increase their sense of personal power? One possibility is that female alcoholics are dealing with the effects of the high frequency of physical and sexual abuse among females (Beckman, 1994a; Swift et al., 1996; Hodgins, El-Guebaly, & Addington, 1997). For example, rates of childhood incest or sexual abuse are much higher among alcoholic women than in alcoholic males or in the general population. Approximately 40 to 75 percent of alcoholic women have experienced rape or incest or both (McDonough & Russell, 1994).

These gender differences in abuse are also found in studies of adolescents. In a sampling from a juvenile detention center, it was found that 46 percent of all subjects reported a history of one or more sexual abuse experiences, 60 percent of the females and 33 percent of the males (Rounds-Bryant, Kristiansen, Fairbank, & Hubbard, 1998). A sample of adolescents from three substance abuse treatment modalities revealed that 25 percent of the females had experienced a form of sexual abuse in the year before treatment, while only 2 percent of the males reported sexual abuse in the previous year (Rounds-Bryant et al., 1998).

In addition, female alcoholics are also more likely than males to report that they were emotionally deprived and unloved as children (McDonough & Russell, 1994). This lack of attachment as a child leads to difficulties in relationships during adolescence, when awkwardness in social skills seems glaringly apparent to peers. This lack of social skills is especially detrimental to girls, whose development is dependent upon a social context.

Such childhood abuse and lack of childhood attachment relationships among female alcoholics may contribute to depression and low self-esteem in females for whom alcohol is used in an effort to increase self-esteem. Research indicates that depression is more common among alcoholic females than among males or the general population (Bushway & Heiland, 1995; Rubin, Stout, & Longabaugh, 1996; Weisner, Mertens, Tam, & Moore, 2001). Depression in females is more likely to be present before the alcohol abuse than after it (Blume, 1998) and may be a predictor of later alcoholism (Nazroo, Edwards, & Brown, 1998). Similarly, research indicates that low self-esteem in junior high school students appears to be a predictor of future alcohol problems for girls but not for boys (Hodgins et al., 1997).

OVERVIEW OF THE RELATIONAL
GROUP THERAPY MODEL

Women's and girls' relationships are essential processes that influence all aspects of female identity, self-concept, and psychological health. Relationships are at the very core of women's identity (Gilligan, 1993). In her research on female development, Gilligan (1993) stressed the inseparable and reciprocal role of relationships and a female's sense of self. Through dynamic social interactions, women and girls create a story of themselves that foretells how they interact with others.

Ideally, girls experience positive and healthy relationships that foster their abilities to nurture both themselves and others. Yet for many of the girls in the juvenile justice system, this ideal never occurs (Calhoun, Bartolumucci, & McLean, in press). Many of their home, school, and even societal contexts are filled with negative forces that are not favorable to the establishment of genuine connections and the development of relational abilities (Miller, 1976). For instance, the majority of female adolescents that are initially involved with juvenile court are charged with offenses such as runaway, truancy, and fornication which are a direct result from relational difficulties with familial, school, and peer relationships (Yates, 1993). Furthermore, it has been found that anywhere between 30 to 70 percent of these girls have experienced sexual abuse (Phelps, McIntosh, Jesudason, Warner, & Pohlkamp, 1982; Finkelhor & Baron, 1986). In addition, it is not unlikely for these girls to have experienced physical abuse or neglect as well as maladaptive home environments (American Correctional Association, 1990).

Lacking meaningful relationships with others, many of these girls develop psychological difficulties or even psychological pathology such as social isolation (Miller, 1976). Delinquency or acting-out behavior is often comorbid with other symptomatology, particularly for females (Miller, Trapani, Fejes-Mendoza, Eggleston, & Dwiggins, 1995). Beginning in adolescence and continuing throughout their lifetimes, females are more likely to experience depression, anxiety, and social stress (Johnson, Roberts, & Worell, 1999). For example, Rutter and Giller (1984) found adolescent girls much more likely to experience depression and suicidal ideation than their male counterparts.

In order to understand the experiences of girls involved in juvenile court, it is essential to have a theoretical means of conceptualizing girls' development and experiences. Numerous researchers in the psychology of women (Miller, 1976; Surrey, 1991; Gilligan, 1993; Brown & Gilligan, 1992) have worked to establish gender-specific theories to better listen to, understand, and conceptualize girls' and women's experiences. A relational model serves to aid in the understanding of the contributing factors in the development of girls who commit aggressive and nonaggressive offenses.

A relational approach views the development of individuals occurring in dynamic relation to essential others. Jordan (1989:1) states, "Viewing development from a relational rather than self perspective, boundaries could be understood as processes of contact and exchange, moments of knowing and movement and growth." Self is defined by Surrey (1991:52) as "a construct useful in describing the organization of a person's experience and construction of reality that illuminates the purpose and directionality of her or his behavior." Gender differences have been noted in how the self is constructed. Miller (1976:83) suggests that a "woman's sense of self becomes very much organized around being able to make and then maintain affiliation and relationships."

Adolescence is a time of psychological and relational crisis for girls, who often become disconnected from themselves and are at an increased risk for depression and trauma (Brown & Gilligan, 1992). Disconnection can occur in interpersonal relationships as well as at the societal level as a consequence of oppression and discrimination. Disconnection at any level hinders or prohibits psychological growth (Jenkins, 1999). Brown and Gilligan (1992), in their continuous exploration of adolescent girls' voices, discovered that many girls discussed a relational crisis in which they felt forced to lose their voice in order to connect with others and maintain relationships. Furthermore, they discovered that women also dissociate from their own adolescent experiences, making it more difficult to understand and recollect the challenges of female adolescence.

IMPLICATIONS FOR TREATMENT: A NEW APPROACH

Given this relational model, treatment programs with females need to address the disconnection with themselves and their relationships. For example, Calhoun (2001) argues that treatment involving females needs to address depression and other internalizing problems. Unfortunately, since most interventions are based on a male model, the majority of treatment programs target externalizing problems. Thus they focus on extinguishing inappropriate behavior while ignoring internalizing problems that females, in particular, may be presenting.

The gender disparities among alcoholics and substance abusers noted earlier need also to be taken into account in the treatment setting. Approaches that focus on females' specific needs are required. For example, we need gender-specific programs (Bushway & Heiland, 1995; Grant, 1997; McDonough & Russell, 1994) that allow for the discussion of gender-specific problems, such as sexual abuse (Rounds-Bryant et al., 1998; Hodgins et al., 1997), in same-gender groups (Hodgins et al., 1997).

In addition, treatment should address the stigma attached to female alcoholism and substance abuse (Beckman, 1994b; Bushway & Heiland, 1995; Kauffman et al., 1997; Rubin et al., 1996; McDonough & Russell, 1994). The perception that female substance abusers are viewed as sexually promiscuous and with low morals not only contributes to decreasing an already lowered level of self-esteem but also keeps many females from seeking treatment (McDonough & Russell, 1994).

Further, when females do seek treatment they often believe that drinking and substance abuse is a symptom of another problem and are more likely to present with a mental health issue or physical complaint (McDonough & Russell, 1994). The mental health issue they are likely to present with is depression, and this needs to be part of an effective treatment plan. Since this depression may be the result of several factors including a history of physical and sexual abuse (Beckman, 1994a; Hodgins et al., 1997; Rounds-Bryant et al., 1998; Swift et al., 1996), low self-esteem (Bushway & Heiland, 1995; Corbin et al., 1997; Hodgins et al., 1997), and gender role conflict (Nazroo et al., 1998) each of these areas needs to be addressed in the treatment process.

Finally, treatment should also take into account females' need for social relationships (Beckman, 1994a; McDonough & Russell, 1994). Understanding the importance of interpersonal relationships in girls' development, group therapy may be a natural way for girls to address problematic issues and foster growth (Butler & Wintram, 1991). Group work provides an opportunity for group members to come together in a therapeutic environment to experience positive and healthy relationships and support from other girls and women (Yalom, 1995).

As girls begin to relate to one another and share themselves in their new relationships, their self-confidence and self-esteem can flourish (Pipher, 1994). Armed with a new sense of self, support, and confidence, the group members can begin to repair the effects of previously harmful relationships and address the hurt, as well as repair the negative consequences of these relationships (Yalom, 1995). Thus working together within a therapeutic group allows diverse girls to come together in a supportive manner to address and challenge their experiences, to develop a sense of female pride, and to create new possibilities for their future (Denmark, 1999). Orenstein (1995:217) has stated, "The most powerful moments of psychological healing and empowerment . . . were those in which, either inadvertently or by design, girls came together to talk about and address experiences of betrayal, unfairness, and hurt."

The primary goals of utilizing a relational group approach with adolescent females involved in juvenile justice is to help them develop positive relationships and healthy connections to foster a sense of support, understanding, and self-pride. The goals for group members are to increase their adaptive skills by enhancing their relational abilities and decreasing their emotional isolation in order to promote psychological health (Brown, 1999).

The group process provides an experience for these girls to come together and confront issues that are common to each of their experiences while creating new opportunities for their futures (Brown,

1999). Way (1995) suggested that decreasing the mistrust, anger, and isolation commonly experienced among these girls can also lead to a decrease in aggression. By improving the relational abilities and confidence of these young women, they will have the knowledge, skills, and experiences to make more positive choices for their futures.

The GIRLS (Gaining Insight into Relationships for Lifelong Success) Project is a gender-specific treatment intervention program that recognizes the central role that relationships play in a female's life. It utilizes the gender-specific relational model previously described. The construction of each session is purposeful. Session content is based upon issues identified in the literature as well as from female juvenile offenders themselves. A description of the content of these sessions may be found in the Appendix.

Supporting Data

Although the relational approach to treating drug and alcohol abuse in female juvenile offenders has been implemented in the GIRLS program, we have only begun gathering data through which to evaluate the effectiveness of this approach. For example, we are beginning to identify some of the factors associated with substance abuse among some of the girls that have participated in the program.

In this initial investigation, the participants were a small sample of female juvenile offenders ($N = 14$) who had completed the Minnesota Multiphasic Personality Inventory–Adolescent (MMPI-A) as part of court-ordered psychological evaluations. These fourteen girls ranged in age from thirteen to seventeen. Eight of the girls were African American and six were Caucasian. These girls tended to be chronic reoffenders whose charges typically included runaway, truancy, unruliness, drug and alcohol offenses, assault, and shoplifting.

In an attempt to identify factors most associated with female substance abuse, we examined a set of preliminary data utilizing the Alcohol/Drug Problem Acknowledgment (ACK) scale of the MMPI-A. This scale was designed to assess the adolescent's willingness to admit to current substance abuse behaviors. The scale consists of thirteen items selected by rational judgment. Almost all the items ask the adolescent to endorse specific behaviors such as drinking alcohol or abusing marijuana, though some items relate more broadly to admitting a willingness to engage in risky or illicit behaviors.

Though the sample size is extremely small and any results are of little practical significance, examination yielded some intriguing results, especially combined with findings from a larger MMPI-A database ($N = 102$) of male offenders. The ACK scale scores for both the sample of females and males were highly correlated with measures of hyperactivity, alienation from self and others, as well as anger and conduct problems. Despite these similarities, the female sample showed a higher relationship between the ACK and the paranoia scale than the males, and a weaker relationship between scores on scales measuring anxiety and family problems and scores on the ACK, than was found with the males. A tentative conclusion from this examination is that male substance abuse may be more related to anxiety, whereas female substance abuse is more related to perceived hostility from others and a distrust of others, while both genders share the common elements of hyperactivity and alienation in association with substance abuse. This provides some support for our perspective that relationships and how the self develops in the context of relationships are of critical importance for girls. Additional data need to be collected, but these preliminary data do point toward females' perception of their relational environment as a hostile place being integral to explaining their substance abuse patterns, whereas males' emotional state, particularly anxiety, may be more pivotal in explaining their substance abuse.

SUMMARY AND CONCLUSIONS

The results we have identified are preliminary and represent a descriptive approach to analysis of the available data. This said, the results are consistent with other research on substance abuse and delinquency in general in that they provide support for the notion that female offending and substance abuse in particular are mediated by both an adolescent's own sense of connection to her family and social environment as well as the degree to which an adolescent experiences anxious and depressive symptoms. The data suggest that there is a particularly strong positive association between high levels of substance abuse and a female adolescent's own sense of bonding and trust with her social support system, particularly her family. Although past research, conducted almost exclusively with males, has pointed toward improving family dynamics, our preliminary data suggest that the sense of connection to one's social support system is an important factor for girls in mediating their involvement in substance abuse. We believe that the relational group therapy model presented here shows great promise in providing an opportunity for girls to recognize and perhaps seek out long-lasting sources of social support.

DISCUSSION QUESTIONS

1. Discuss how Calhoun, Stefurak, and Johnson outline the key differences between males and females when it comes to reasons for drinking and the implications of these differences for effective treatment of female alcoholics.
2. The *relational group therapy* model proposed here by the authors is yet another example of the typical group counseling approach to substance abuse treatment. How does what they propose here differ from other group counseling models, some of which have been described in other chapters in this text?
3. Do the preliminary findings presented by the authors support their overall recommendation that relational group therapy, as they describe it here, be used with the female substance-addicted offender? Explain.

APPENDIX:
GIRLS (GAINING INSIGHT INTO RELATIONSHIPS FOR LIFELONG SUCCESS) PROJECT MODULES

Purpose

- To become aware of healthy alternatives to their current offending behaviors
- To make healthier decisions that will promote positive self-concept and relationships
- To increase their adaptive skills necessary to create and fulfill future goals
- To foster a sense of social belonging as contributing members of their community

Sessions 1 and 2: Joining

- To develop a trusting relationship between group facilitators and participants
- To create a positive and empowering, rather than delinquent, identity among group members
- To foster a sense of belonging to the group through the creation of a group name and statement of purpose
- To establish rules, boundaries, rights, and responsibilities for group participation

Sessions 3 and 4: Educational/Vocational Goals

- To utilize career assessment tools to help girls become aware of the numerous vocational opportunities available to them
- To help girls identify areas of strength and interest
- To encourage the girls' involvement in prosocial activities

Sessions 5 and 6: Substance Abuse

- To explore the patterns of substance abuse within their families
- To increase their understanding of drugs and alcohol and their recognition of the short- and long-term consequences of using drugs and alcohol
- To heighten their awareness of how drugs and alcohol decrease their ability to engage in prosocial activities and positive decision making, as well as how drugs and alcohol perpetuate feelings of low self-worth
- To help girls identify the underlying causes of their needs to abuse substances and to find healthier alternatives to dealing with these issues

Sessions 7 and 8: Anger and Violence

- To recognize the patterns of anger and violence within their interpersonal relationships
- To identify feelings of anger and recognize their unhealthy means of dealing with anger through violence and offending behaviors
- To explore both positive and negative means of expressing anger and increase their skill to deal with anger in a constructive manner

Sessions 9 and 10: Sexuality

- To increase their awareness of the societal gender prescriptions
- To empower girls to take control over their bodies and learn positive means of expressing their desires
- To process events of sexual coercion and abuse experienced and discuss possible means of protection against future victimization

Sessions 11 and 12: Pregnancy/Motherhood

- To dispel myths of contraception and empower girls to take responsibility for their sexual behaviors
- To explore the appeal of motherhood and to find alternate means to fulfill the emotional needs, such as love, connection, and purpose, that lead to adolescent motherhood
- To recognize how pregnancy as an adolescent can influence their lifelong decisions and opportunities
- To help pregnant girls and adolescent mothers become connected with services and resources to help them with their parenting skills as well as support them in the achievement of their goals

Sessions 13 and 14: Grief and Loss

- To identify and process experienced losses associated with the absence of family members, suicide, and miscarriages/abortions and loss that has occurred as a result of violence
- To explore the emotional (shame, guilt, depression) and behavioral consequences (offending behavior) associated with grief and loss
- To foster strength and resiliency through helping girls develop social support networks to deal more openly with their multiple losses

Sessions 15 and 16: New Beginnings

- To summarize new possibilities and alternative means to offending behaviors
- To discuss ways they have committed to engaging in prosocial behaviors
- To process the meaning of belonging to a group with shared goals and common experiences
- To discuss the feelings associated with belonging to a group that supports personal growth and encourages their involvement and abilities to engage in numerous opportunities for their future

REFERENCES

American Correctional Association. (1990). *The female offender: What does the future hold?* Washington, DC: St. Mary's Press.

Bartolomucci, C. (2002). Does nature of offense matter? An examination of psychological and relationship factors between aggressive and non-aggressive female juvenile offenders. Unpublished doctoral dissertation, University of Georgia.

Beckman, L. (1994a). Barriers to alcoholism treatment for women. *Alcohol Health & Research World, 18*(3), 208.

Beckman, L. (1994b). Treatment needs of women with alcohol problems. *Alcohol Health & Research World, 18,* 206-216.

Blume, S. (1998). Alcoholism in women. *Harvard Mental Health Letter, 14*(9), 5-8.

Brown, L. (1999). The others in my I: Adolescent girls' friendships and peer relations. In N. Johnson, M. Roberts, & J. Worell (Eds.), *Beyond appearance: A new look at adolescent girls* (pp. 377-404). Washington, DC: American Psychological Association.

Brown, L. & Gilligan, D.C. (1992). *Meeting at the crossroads: Women's psychology and girls' development.* Cambridge, MA: Harvard University Press.

Bushway, D. & Heiland, L. (1995). Women in treatment for addiction: What's new in the literature? *Alcoholism Treatment Quarterly, 13*(4), 83-96.

Butler, S. & Wintram, C. (1991). *Feminist groupwork.* Thousand Oaks, CA: Sage.

Calhoun, G.B. (2001). An examination of behavioral and emotional differences between male and female juvenile offenders. *Journal of Offender Rehabilitation, 33*(2), 87-96.

Calhoun, G.B., Bartolomucci, C., & McLean, B. (in press). Building connections: Relational group work with female adolescent offenders. *Women & Therapy.*

Calhoun, G.B., Glaser, B.A., & Bartolomucci, C.L. (1999). Counseling the juvenile offender. In A.M. Horne & M.S. Kiselica (Eds.), *Handbook of counseling boys and adolescent males: A practitioner's guide* (pp. 131-141). Thousand Oaks, CA: Sage.

Chesney-Lind, M. & Sheldon, R. (1998). *Girls, delinquency, and juvenile justice* (2nd rev.). Albany, NY: Wadsworth.

Corbin, W., McNair, L., & Carter, J. (1996). Self-esteem and problem drinking among male and female college students. *Journal of Alcohol and Drug Education, 42,* 1-14.

Denmark, F. (1999). Enhancing the development of adolescent girls. In N. Johnson, M. Roberts, & J. Worell (Eds.), *Beyond appearance: A new look at adolescent girls* (pp. 377-404). Washington, DC: American Psychological Association.

Finklehor, D. & Baron, L. (1986). Risk factors for child sexual abuse. *Journal of Interpersonal Violence, 1,* 43-71.

Gilligan, C. (1993). *In a different voice: Psychological theory and women's development.* Cambridge, MA: Harvard University Press.

Grant, B. (1997). Barriers to alcoholism treatment: Reasons for not seeking treatment in a general population sample. *Journal of Studies on Alcohol, 58*(4), 365-371.

Hodgins, D., El-Guebaly, N., & Addington, J. (1997). Treatment of substance abusers: Single or mixed gender programs? *Addiction, 92*(7), 805-812.

Jenkins, Y. (1999). The Stone Center theoretical approach revisited: Applications for African American women. In L. Jackson & B. Greene (Eds.), *Psychotherapy with African American women: Innovations in psychodynamic perspectives and practice* (pp. 62-81). New York: Guilford.

Johnson, N.G., Roberts, M.C., & Worell, J. (1999). *Beyond appearance: A look at adolescent girls.* Washington, DC: American Psychological Association.

Jordan, J. (1989). Relational development: Therapeutic implications of empathy and shame. Work in progress, No. 39. Wellesley, MA: Stone Center Working Paper Series.

Kauffman, S., Silver, P., & Poulin, J. (1997). Gender differences in attitudes toward alcohol, tobacco, and other drugs. *Social Work, 42*(3), 231-241.

McDonough, R. & Russell, L. (1994). Alcoholism in women: A holistic, comprehensive care model. *Journal of Mental Health Counseling, 16*(4), 459-474.

Miller, D., Trapani, C., Fejes-Mendoza, K., Eggleston, C., & Dwiggins, D. (1995). Adolescent female offenders: Unique considerations. *Adolescence, 30*(118), 429-434.

Miller, J.B. (1976). *Toward a new psychology of women.* Boston: Beacon Press.

Nazroo, J., Edwards, A., & Brown, G. (1998). Gender differences in the prevalence of depression: Artifacts, alternative disorders, biology or roles? *Sociology of Health & Illness, 20*(3), 312-330.

Orenstein, P. (1995). *School girls: Young women, self-esteem, and the confidence gap.* New York: Doubleday.

Phelps, R.J., McIntosh, M., Jesudason, V., Warner, P., & Pohlkamp, J. (1982). *Wisconsin Juvenile Offender Project.* Madison: Youth Policy and Law Center, Wisconsin Council on Juvenile Justice.

Pipher, M. (1994). *Reviving Ophelia: Saving the selves of adolescent girls.* New York: Ballantine Books.

Rounds-Bryant, J., Kristiansen, P., Fairbank, J., & Hubbard, R. (1998). Substance use, mental disorders, abuse, and crime: Gender comparisons among a national sample of adolescent drug treatment clients. *Journal of Child & Adolescent Substance Abuse, 7*(4), 19-34.

Rubin, A., Stout, R., & Longabaugh, R. (1996). Gender differences in relapse situations. *Addiction, 91*(Supplement), S111-S120.

Rutter, M. & Giller, H. (1984). *Juvenile delinquency: Trends and perspectives.* New York: Guilford Press.

Stone, S.S. (1998). Changing the nature of juvenile offenders. Available at <http://ojjdp.ncjrs.org/conference/track1.html>.

Surrey, J. (1991). The self-in-relation: A theory of women's development. In J. Jordan, J. Baker Miller, I. Stiver, & J. Surrey (Eds.), *Women's growth in connection: Writings from the Stone Center* (pp. 51-66). New York: Guilford Press.

Swift, W., Copeland, J., & Hall, W. (1996). Characteristics of women with alcohol and other drug problems: Findings of an Australian national survey. *Addiction, 91*(8), 1141-1151.

Thombs, D. (1993). The differentially discriminating properties of alcohol expectancies for female and male drinkers. *Journal of Counseling & Development, 71*(3), 321-325.

Way, N.E. (1995). "Can't you see the courage, the strength that I have?" Listening to urban adolescent girls speak about their relationship. *Psychology of Women Quarterly, 19,* 107-128.

Weisner, C., Mertens, J., Tam, T., & Moore, C. (2001). Factors affecting the initiation of substance abuse treatment in managed care. *Addiction, 96,* 705-716.

Yalom, I. (1995). *The theory and practice of group psychotherapy* (4th ed.). New York: Basic Books.

Yates, A. (1993). Issues of autonomy in adolescence: The "superwoman." In M. Sugar (Ed.), *Female adolescent development* (pp. 57-167). New York: Brunner/Mazel Publishers.

Chapter 12

Assessing Program Needs of Female Offenders Who Abuse Substances

Dawn Marie Baletka
Robert A. Shearer

The number of individuals being incarcerated in criminal justice facilities, particularly female offenders, in the United States has experienced a tremendous increase (Farabee et al., 1999; Peugh & Belenko, 1999). Much of this increase can be attributed to (1) the commitment of law enforcement personnel to take a strict stance on the arrest and prosecution of drug-related offenses and to (2) mandatory sentences (Bloom, Chesney-Lind, & Owen, 1994; Collins & Collins, 1996; Farabee et al., 1999; Peugh & Belenko, 1999). According to the Federal Bureau of Prisons (1997), drug offenders accounted for 6 percent (19,000) of the state prison population in 1980 and 21 percent (236,800) of the state prison population in 1998. The increase was just as dramatic in the federal prison populations, which indicate that 25 percent (4,749) of the population had drug offenses in 1980, while 59 percent (55,984) had drug offenses in 1998. The Center on Addiction and Substance Abuse (1998) claims that approximately 80 percent of state and federal inmates (1) committed offenses under the influence of drugs or alcohol at the time of their crime, (2) committed their crime to support their drug use, or (3) had histories of problematic substance use. Thus it is clear that substance abuse among inmate populations has increased to the point where criminal justice facilities are finding themselves searching for ways to keep pace with treatment options.

This is especially true for the female inmate population. The number of female inmates has risen 336 percent since 1980, whereas the number of male inmates has increased at 189 percent (Maguire & Pastore, 1997). This has led to women entering substance abuse treatment in increasing numbers and a greater proportion coming to treatment through the criminal justice system rather than from any other avenue (Institute of Medicine, 1990). However, this dramatic increase in female offenders does not coincide with an equivalent increase in female prison facilities or rehabilitation/treatment programs geared toward the needs of female offenders.

The correctional system has historically been male dominated (Clement, 1997). The structure of prison settings, the rules, the operating procedures, and the treatment programs are largely based not only on the needs of males but also on research studying the effectiveness of programs based on male subjects. Correctional systems are frequently able to assign male inmates to facilities based on the individual rehabilitative or treatment needs of the offender, the severity of the crime the offender committed, and/or the security risk of the offender (Clement, 1997).

Female inmates are not afforded these same considerations. Prison facilities that house female offenders are few in number. Most states within the United States have only one facility to house female inmates (Clement, 1997). Thus most female offenders are assigned to facilities not based on their individual rehabilitative or treatment needs, issues of security, or the severity of the offense committed, but on the sole basis of gender. This is true even though female offenders who abuse drugs are the fastest-growing segment of the criminal justice system (Wellisch, Prendergast, & Anglin, 1994).

ASSESSMENT AND TREATMENT PROGRAMS IN THE CORRECTIONAL ENVIRONMENT

Because standard treatment modalities are almost exclusively male dominated in content and structure, most prison facilities are ill prepared to offer women gender-specific treatment and aftercare programming. Women with substance abuse problems have specific needs and concerns that are not addressed in standard treatment settings.

Many correctional treatment programs do not assess the multiple problems of substance-abusing female offenders (Covington, 2000; Peugh & Belenko, 1999). Female offenders with substance abuse problems are often placed into treatment programs that are based on male needs (See Table 12.1). However, female substance abusers have needs that are very much different from those of their male counterparts (Peugh & Belenko, 1999). It is important that the needs of individuals with substance abuse problems be addressed in gender-appropriate ways (Peugh & Belenko, 1999).

Both male and female substance abusers experience compounding mental health problems (Alexander, Craig, MacDonald, & Haugland, 1994; Helzer & Pryzbeck, 1988; McCarty, Argeriou, Huebner, & Lubran, 1991; Regier et al., 1990; Teplin, Abram, & McClelland, 1996; Wilcox & Yates, 1993). However, female substance abusers experience different types of mental health problems than do males. Females in correctional facilities have a history of experiencing physical, sexual, and psychological abuse at higher rates than males (Cosden & Cortez-Ison, 1998; Gomberg & Nirenberg, 1993; Wellisch, Anglin,

TABLE 12.1. Paradigm of substance abuse: Female versus male treatment

Treatment	Male	Female
Vocational training	Effective	Highly effective
Parenting skills	Low motivation/high resistance	High motivation/low resistance
Family therapy	Low need	High need
Mental health	Substance abuse, antisocial, psychosis, personality disorders	Substance abuse, depression, post-traumatic stress (childhood abuse)
High-risk behaviors	Intravenous drug use, sexual activities without condoms	Intravenous drug use, sexual activities without condoms, sex for money or drugs, partner with substance use problem
HIV/AIDS	Moderate risk factor	High-risk factor
Confrontational techniques	Effective	Limited effectiveness
Anger management	Effective	Limited effectiveness
Group therapy	Moderately effective	Very limited effectiveness
Individual therapy	Effective	Effective
Empowerment training	Limited need	Highly effective

& Prendergast, 1993; Institute of Medicine, 1990). They also are more likely than men to use drugs and alcohol as a coping mechanism for traumatic events and stress (Peugh & Belenko, 1999; Falkin et al., 1994; Griffin, Weiss, Mirin, & Lang, 1989; Hser, Anglin, & Booth, 1987; McClellan, Farabee, & Crouch, 1997). The differences in the mental health problems between males and females, and the circumstances that precipitate drug and alcohol use, need to be confronted in substance abuse treatment using different interventions and auxiliary services.

Hartel (1994) discussed that women who are intraveneous drug users are more likely than male injection drug users (IDUs) to engage in high-risk sex with multiple partners, to exchange sex for money or drugs, to share needles, and to engage in unprotected sex with other IDUs. These behaviors lead to an increased risk of contracting a sexually transmitted disease (STD). Untreated STDs in women are likely to lead to serious health complications such as pelvic inflammatory disease (PID), cervical cancer, and infertility. Furthermore, untreated STDs are associated with increased rates of HIV transmission (Eng & Butler, 1996; McCoy, Miles, & Inciardi, 1995).

HIV and AIDS are crucial issues for substance-involved female inmates. The number of HIV-positive female state inmates increased 88 percent between 1991 and 1995. In contrast, the number of HIV-positive male state inmates increased by 28 percent during the same time frame (Maruschak, 1997). HIV infection rates among females are predominantly related to injecting drugs, engaging in sexual activities with IDUs, using crack cocaine, and participating in unsafe sexual practices such as unprotected sex and prostitution for drugs (Centers for Disease Control and Prevention, 1996; Inciardi, Lockwood, & Pottieger, 1993; McCoy et al., 1995). Thus female substance users have a great need for safe-sex education.

For female inmates, HIV education and prevention skills are an essential part of substance abuse treatment because the knowledge of the consequences of drug use and the skills necessary to protect themselves against the transmission of HIV is vital. These skills include negotiating with partners to use condoms and asking partners about their sexual and injection drug use histories (Peugh & Belenko, 1999).

Treatment Techniques and Program Designs

The use of confrontational techniques and group settings, typically used in treatment models for men, are routinely not effective for women (Kelly, Kropp, & Manhal-Baugus, 1995; Ramsey, 1980). Confrontational treatment models tend to be threatening to many women and often inhibit the ability of female substance abusers to address the underlying factors of their addiction (Peugh & Belenko, 1999). Some of these factors include physical and sexual abuse, feelings of worthlessness, and an extreme desire to please others.

Programs for men also often include anger-management training to promote appropriate means of expressing anger. Women, however, are more likely to have trouble expressing anger in any form (Inciardi et al., 1993) and would be much better served with alternative skills training. Women tend to respond more positively to treatment that includes techniques which reduce feelings of guilt and self-blame and improve self-esteem and self-awareness (Covington, 1998; Wells & Jackson, 1992).

Male treatment programs rarely address issues involving parenting training. Females are more receptive to parenting-skills training within the treatment process than are men, and thus this type of programming is essential for female inmates (Peugh & Belenko, 1999). Correctional Care (1994) reported that 50 to 70 percent of incarcerated females had one or more children living with them at the time of their imprisonment. Females tend to be the primary caregivers of children. Alcohol and drug abuse has been cited as a causative factor in up to 80 percent of substantiated cases of child abuse and neglect (Azzi-Lessing & Olsen, 1996). Parenting groups have been shown to be highly successful with recovering addicts (Plasse, 1995). A majority of these women claimed that parenting-skills classes were "very important" to their treatment program.

Male substance abusers often come from families who abuse drugs and alcohol; however, family issues are rarely brought forth in counseling sessions. Female substance users are even more likely than males to come from drug- and alcohol-abusive families (Marsh & Miller, 1985). An increasing amount of evidence suggests that women with substance abuse problems frequently have a childhood trauma that may be an important contributing factor to their addictive behavior (Janikowski & Glover, 1994). Family interventions, which are rarely used in correctional facilities (Liddle & Dakof, 1995), have been shown to be effective even when the entire family does not participate (Barber & Gilbertson, 1997; Szapocznik, Kurtines, Foote, Perez-Vidal, & Hervis, 1983).

Vocational and educational programs are readily available to men in substance abuse treatment. The programs offered are traditional male roles in society and allow them to learn a trade that pays a living wage when they reenter society if they so choose. However, female substance abusers receive very little vocational and educational training (Gray, Mays, & Stoher, 1995). The training that they do receive is typically for low-paying jobs with little opportunity for advancement. Most female offenders who are also mothers expect to return to their children after release from the correctional facility. Many of these women do not expect to receive financial or emotional support from their children's father (Prendergast, Wellisch, & Falkin, 1995). Without a marketable skill and the ability to use socially acceptable interpersonal skills, a large majority of female inmates will reoffend (Shearer & Baletka, 1999). Vocational and educational training for incarcerated females enables them to obtain jobs that provide a living wage, thus allowing them to be actively involved in raising their children.

THE DEVELOPMENT OF GENDER-SPECIFIC SUBSTANCE ABUSE PROGRAMS

There are existing substance abuse programs and curricula in correctional literature and practice, but few of these programs are gender specific and empirically supported. Several sources in the literature about female offenders have indicated the importance of various curriculum areas in correctional programs. The Center for Substance Abuse Treatment (1994), for example, identified seventeen issues that needed to be addressed in a comprehensive treatment program for women. These issues ranged from gender-specific addiction issues to child care and custody, including interpersonal violence, relationships with family members, and low self-esteem. Covington (1999), in reviewing the seventeen issues in the Center for Substance Abuse report, concluded that professionals and recovering women agreed on the issues most central to recovery. These issues fell into four categories: self, relationships, sexuality, and spirituality. These four issues serve as the foundation for her four treatment modules in a comprehensive program for use in the criminal justice system. Her treatment program is widely accepted and professionally constructed, but it is not clear how a program assesses needs using her treatment modules. Crowe and Reeves (1994) suggest needs assessments that address physical and sexual abuse, including incest. Vigdal (1995) recognizes including all of these in needs assessment and adds issues associated with housing needs, vocational training, and medical services.

Drabble (1996) completed an extensive overview of elements of effective services for women in substance abuse treatment. She identified several service areas which included medical health care issues, emotional/psychological issues, life skills training, partner and parenting issues, and cultural/population-specific services.

The focus of this chapter is a demonstration of how one curricula component of a program designed to ensure that programming is meeting identified goals of treatment for female clients could be used in other ways by correctional managers. The development of a multiple-use instrument is discussed next, along with a discussion of issues of reliability and validity. The chapter concludes with further discussion of how the use of the instrument can benefit correctional managers and program providers who are providing substance abuse treatment to the female correctional client.

The Female Offender Critical Intervention Inventory

The Female Offender Critical Intervention Inventory (FOCI) was developed by drawing on the accepted issue areas in the field and by careful testing of the internal reliability and validity of the instrument, drawing heavily on the efforts by Sanders, McNeill, Rienzi, and DeLouth (1997). With minor modifications, the eighteen items in their survey that were rated with the highest level of importance were selected for reliability and validity testing in the current study. These items are scored on a three-point scale (never = 0; sometimes = 1; frequently = 2), with a range of zero to thirty-six. A high score on the scale indicates that clients are indeed being asked about problems that have been found to be highly concentrated among female substance abusers, and a low score on the items indicates that program staff are not sufficiently addressing these issues with their clients. A description of those items included in the FOCI instrument are addressed further in the following sections and in Table 12.2.

THE PRESENT STUDY

The FOCI inventory was administered to four groups of female felony offenders in four units of a prison system in the southwestern United States. All participants were selected by directors of the substance abuse programs based on availability at the time of the testing. Participants were instructed prior to the survey that participation was voluntary and anonymous. The survey was read aloud to all groups. Group 1 consisted of fifty-two adult female offenders in a state jail, and group 2 consisted of fifty-two adult female offenders in a substance abuse felony punishment facility. Group 3 consisted of fifty-two adult female offenders in a privately contracted therapeutic community (TC), and group 4 consisted of thirty-two female offenders in a prison-based therapeutic community.

DATA ANALYSIS AND FINDINGS

A priori assumptions about the possibility that the eighteen FOCI items could be broken out into several basic underlying theoretical constructs called for a testing of those assumptions using a data reduction technique. We conducted a series of factor analytic techniques to get a first look at which of the items included in the analysis could be viewed as measuring the same concept. This is important because it gives treatment providers a clearer understanding of the theory behind the questions being posed which, in turn, can be connected more closely with the treatment practices that have been designed based on the major concepts associated with explanations for why people abuse substances.

As shown in Table 12.2, the eighteen questions from the FOCI instrument loaded on three separate factors, with the lowest factor loading (.33) for the item "My counselor or group has talked with me about emotional abuse of me and others around me." This is still within the acceptable range since much of the literature suggests that for the development of new scales, factor loadings of .35 or higher are acceptable (Sims, 2003; Hair, Anderson, Tatham, & Black, 1992;

TABLE 12.2. FOCI factor analysis

Factor	Questions	Factor loadings
Substance abuse— lifestyle risk	Q6: My counselor or group has talked with me about dependency problems.	.82
	Q7: AIDS awareness has been discussed with me by my counselor or group.	.60
	Q8: My counselor or group has talked with me about lifestyle alternatives to drug abuse and addiction.	.68
	Q13: My counselor has talked with me about the process of recovery from drugs or alcohol.	.68
	Q18: My counselor or group has discussed with me problems with alcohol dependency.	.70
	Q9: Violence in relationships has been discussed with me by my counselor or group.	.53
Abuse	QI: My counselor or group has talked to me about physical abuse as a child.	.83
	Q2: My counselor or group has talked to me about childhood sexual abuse.	.78
	Q11: Stress and temptation has been discussed with me by my counselor or group.	.44
	Q12: My counselor or group has talked with me about emotional abuse of me and others around me.	.33
	Q14: Sexual abuse has been discussed with me by my counselor or group.	.69
Personal attribute	Q4: My counselor or group has talked with me about my self-esteem.	.63
	Q5: My counselor or group has talked with me about treatment programs available to me.	.52
	Q15: Skills have been discussed with me by my counselor or group.	.52

TABLE 12.2 *(continued)*

Factor	Questions	Factor loadings
	Q16: Anger management has been discussed with me by my counselor or group.	.96
	Q17: Becoming an alcohol or drug counselor has been discussed with me by my counselor or group.	.71
No identifiable factor	Q3: My counselor or group has talked with me about the effects of addiction on a parent.	
	Q10: My counselor or group has talked with me about physical abuse of others in my family.	

Rossi, Wright, & Anderson, 1983). The additional factor loadings ranged from .44 to .96. As noted in Table 12.2, two of the FOCI items did not load on any underlying theorectical dimension and were therefore discarded.

Based on the theorectical constructs associated with the grouped FOCI items, the three factors that emerged from the factor analysis were labeled substance abuse and lifestyle risk, abuse, and personal attributes. As shown in Table 12.2, the six questions that loaded on the substance abuse and lifestyle risk factor all appear to be addressing problems directly associated with substance abuse (Q6, Q13, Q18) or with lifestyle risks for substance abuse (Q7, Q8, Q9). The five questions that loaded on the abuse factor all address some type of abuse, with the exception of Q11. This question addresses the issue of stress and its involvement in the temptation to use substances as a way of escaping those situations that produce it. It could be that individuals view abuse as a major stressor when it comes to "escapist" behavior through the use of substances and so identified it here as being part and parcel of the abuse dimension.

The third factor, personal attributes, is composed of five questions, all of which appear to be providing possible solutions to the problems that many substance-abusing females are found to be in dire need of understanding. Self-esteem issues (Q4), basic social and self-efficacy skills training (Q15), and coming to grips with managing anger (Q16) are all crucial components to substance abuse treatment programs, especially for the female correctional client as has been discussed in previous chapters. Becoming aware of the type of treatment that is available (Q5) coupled with the empowering tool of oneself becoming a substance abuse counselor (Q17) are equally important for this particular client.

Subsequent Data Analysis

Based on the findings from the factor analysis, and after further review, fifteen items were used to develop three separate scales that could be used in subsequent data analysis and that more clearly represent the three identified underlying theoretical constructs. Question 9 was excluded because it did not seem to be theoretically linked to the other questions included in that initial factor. Recall from Table 12.2 that it in fact addresses the issue of violence in relationships and would have seemed to be a better fit for the abuse factor. Consequently, the revised scales can be seen to reliably address those problem areas that have been found to be directly related to the abuse of substances by females. These three areas are similar to those identified earlier by Covington (1999), although they are missing the issue of spirituality, a key area for females as indicated by that particular study.

Use of the FOCI Scales for Corrections

Shearer and Baletka (2000) first developed the FOCI questionnaire as part of a treatment program curricula that would measure the extent to which clients were actually receiving information about those issues identified in the literature as being associated with substance abuse by females. Here we tested the reliability and validity of that eighteen-item instrument, finding it to represent three underlying theoretical constructs. We further indicate that because the factor analysis proved successful at identifying those constructs, three separate scales could be developed and used as indices in future programming and/or research. In particular, we suggest that the FOCI instrument could be used to evaluate the extent to which programs are adequately addressing with clients these important issues related to their everyday lives. To reiterate yet again, this instrument was created drawing from the literature and the myriad of studies that have examined the reasons why females abuse substances. It is, therefore, one that receives high marks for construct validity.

Further, by changing the wording of the questions, the FOCI instrument could also be used as a reliable and valid assessment tool during the intake process of female correctional clients. For example, Q4, "My counselor or group has talked with me about my self-esteem," could be changed to "I would like for my counselor or group to talk with me about my self-esteem." Although we recognize that further testing of the reliability and validity of such a changed instrument is certainly called for, we believe this is a step in the right direction.

One final use of the FOCI instrument could be to guide corrections managers and treatment providers in curriculum development. A program that is grounded in sound theory and empirical testing is, after all, much more likely to succeed at reducing relapse and thus prolonging recovery than a program that is not.

SUMMARY AND CONCLUSIONS

Effective treatment strategies for female offenders include comprehensive approaches. These comprehensive approaches include individual counseling, group counseling, vocational training, parenting training, long-term refusal and resistance skills training, and education on safe sex and domestic violence (Peugh & Belenko, 1999; Shearer & Baletka, 1999). The FOCI-R is an example of an assessment tool that can help improve the effectiveness of treatment programs by viewing curriculums through the eyes of the client, thus helping program administrators to provide more comprehensive services. The results of correctional-based substance abuse treatment research suggest that well-designed, gender-specific programs of sufficient length which are linked to aftercare services in the community can reduce post-release criminal activity, relapse, and recidivism.

Much more needs to be done to ensure that substance abuse programming in all areas and for all types of clients (males, females, juveniles, etc.) is meeting the goal of producing substance-free individuals. But the work that is underway in this area of correctional programming has come a long way from the earlier days of attributing substance abuse to a mere personal and criminal problem. The treatment community has recognized that what works for male correctional clients will not work for females, and findings such as those presented here certainly do provide promising directions for future development of more comprehensive programming as well as the measures that can be used to evaluate them.

DISCUSSION QUESTIONS

1. Discuss the policy implications of the FOCI instrument as outlined by Baletka and Shearer.
2. Generally speaking, describe the special needs of female substance abusers using the three underlying dimensions produced by the authors' statistical analysis.
3. Think about how what Baletka and Shearer proposed here could be used in conjunction with those findings and subsequent suggestions for treating the female substance-abusing correctional client discussed in Chapter 11.

REFERENCES

Alexander, M.J., Craig, T.L., MacDonald, J., & Haugland, G. (1994). Dual diagnosis in a state psychiatric facility. *American Journal of Addiction, 3*(4), 314-324.

Azzi-Lessing, L. & Olsen, L.J. (1996). Substance abuse-affected families in the child welfare system: New challenges, new alliances. *Social Work, 4*(1), 15-23.

Barber, J.G. & Gilbertson, R. (1997). Unilateral interventions for women living with heavy drinkers. *Social Work, 42*(1), 69-78.

Bloom, B., Chesney-Lind, M., & Owen, B. (1994). *Women in California prisons: Hidden victims of the war on drugs.* San Francisco: Center on Juvenile and Criminal Justice.

Center for Substance Abuse Treatment. (1994). *Practical approaches in the treatment of women who abuse alcohol and other drugs.* Rockville, MD: Department of Health and Human Services, Public Health Service.

Center on Addiction and Substance Abuse. (1998). *Behind bars: Substance abuse and America's prison population.* New York: Columbia University Press.

Centers for Disease Control and Prevention, Center for Infectious Diseases, Division of HIV/AIDS, National Center for Infectious Diseases, and Division of HIV/AIDS. (1996). U.S. HIV and AIDS cases reported through December 1996. HIV/AIDS Surveillance Report No. 8. Atlanta, GA: Authors.

Clement, M. (1997). New treatment for drug abusing women offenders in Virginia. *Journal of Offender Rehabilitation, 25*(1-2), 61-81.

Collins, W. & Collins, A. (1996). *Women in jail: Legal issues.* Washington, DC: National Institute of Corrections.

Correctional Care. (1994, December). National commission issues, position statement on women's health. Washington, DC: National Institute of Justice.

Cosden, M. & Cortez-Ison, E. (1998). Sexual abuse, parental bonding, social support, and program retention for women in substance abuse treatment. *Journal of Substance Abuse Treatment, 16*(2), 149-155.

Covington, S.S. (1998). Women in prison: Approaches in the treatment of our most invisible population. In J. Harden & M. Hill (Eds.), *Breaking the rules: Women in prison and feminist therapy* (pp. 141-145). Binghamton, NY: The Haworth Press.

Covington, S.S. (1999). *Helping women recover: A program for treating substance abuse addiction.* San Francisco: Harper.

Covington, S.S. (2000). Helping women recover creating gender-specific treatment for substance-abusing women and girls in community corrections. In M. McMahon (Ed.), *Assessment to assistance: Programs for women in community corrections* (pp. 171-233). Lanham, MD: American Correctional Association.

Crowe, A.H. & Reeves, R. (1994). *Treatment for alcohol and other drug abuse; TAP 11.* Rockville, MD: Center for Substance Abuse Treatment, U.S. Department of Health and Human Services.

Drabble, L. (1996). Elements of effective services for women in recovery: Implications for clinicians and program supervisors. In B.L. Underhill & G.G. Finnegan (Eds.), *Chemical dependency: Women at risk* (pp. 1-21). Binghamton, NY: The Haworth Press.

Eng, T. & Butler, W. (Eds.). (1996). *The hidden epidemic: Confronting sexually transmitted diseases.* Washington, DC: National Academy Press.

Falkin, G.P., Wellisch, J., Prendergast, M.L., Killian, T., Hawke, J., Natarajan, M., Kowalewski, M., & Owens, B. (1994). *Drug treatment for women offenders: A systems perspective.* Washington, DC: U.S. Department of Justice.

Farabee, D., Prendergast, M., Cartier, J., Wexler, H., Knight, K., & Anglin, M.D. (1999). Barriers to implementing effective correctional drug treatment programs. *The Prison Journal, 79*(2), 150-162.

Federal Bureau of Prisons, U.S. Department of Justice (1997). *Federal Bureau of Prisons quick facts.* Washington, DC: Office of Justice Programs.

Gomberg, E.S.L. & Nirenberg, T.D. (1993). Antecedents and consequences. In E.S.L. Goldberg & T.D. Nirenberg (Eds.), *Women and substance abuse* (pp. 118-141). Norwood, NJ: Ablex Publishing Co.

Gray, T., Mays, G.L., & Stoher, M.K. (1995). Inmate needs and programming in exclusively women's jails. *The Prison Journal, 75,* 186-202.

Griffin, M.L., Weiss, R.D., Mirin, S.M., & Lang, U. (1989). A comparison of male and female cocaine abusers. *Archives of General Psychiatry, 46,* 122-126.

Hair, J.F., Anderson, R.E., Tatham, R.L., & Black, W.C. (1992). *Multivariate data analysis* (3rd ed.). New York: Macmillan Publishing.

Hartel, D. (1994). Context of HIV risk behavior among female injecting drug users and female sexual partners of injecting drug users. In R. Battjes, A. Sloboda, & W. Grace (Eds.), *The context of risk among drug users and their sexual partners* (pp. 41-47). NIDA Research Monograph No. 143. Bethesda, MD: National Institute on Drug Abuse, National Institute of Health.

Helzer, J.E. & Pryzbeck, T.R. (1988). The co-occurrence of alcoholism with other psychiatric disorders in the general population and its impact on treatment. *Journal of Studies on Alcohol, 49,* 219-224.

Hser, Y., Anglin, M.D., & Booth, M.W. (1987). Sex differences in addict careers. *American Journal of Drug and Alcohol Abuse, 13,* 231-251.

Inciardi, J.A., Lockwood, D., & Pottieger, A.E. (1993). *Women and crack cocaine.* New York: Macmillian.

Institute of Medicine. (1990). *Treating drug problems* (Vol. 1). Washington, DC: National Academy Press.

Janikowski, T.P. & Glover, N. (1994). Incest and substance abuse: Implications for treatment professionals. *Journal of Substance Abuse Treatment, 11*(3), 177-183.

Kelly, V., Kropp, F.B., & Manhal-Baugus, M. (1995). The association of program-related variables to length of sobriety: A pilot study of chemically dependent women. *Journal of Addictions and Offender Counseling, 15,* 42-50.

Liddle, J.A. & Dakof, G.A. (1995). Efficacy of family therapy for drug abuse: Promising but not definitive. *Journal of Marital and Family Therapy, 21,* 511-543.

Maguire, K. & Pastore, A.L. (1997). *Sourcebook of criminal justice statistics.* Washington, DC: U.S. Department of Justice.

Marsh, J.C. & Miller, N.A. (1985). Female clients in substance abuse treatment. *International Journal of Addiction, 20*(6-7), 995-1019.

Maruschak, L. (1997). *HIV in prisons and jails, 1995.* Bureau of Justice Statistics Bulletin. Washington, DC: U.S. Department of Justice.

McCarty, D.S., Argeriou, M., Huebner, R.B., & Lubran, B. (1991). Alcoholism, drug abuse and the homeless. *American Psychologist, 46,* 1139-1148.

McClellan, D.S., Farabee, D., & Crouch, B.M. (1997). Early victimization, drug use, and criminality: A comparison of male and female prisoners. *Criminal Justice and Behavior, 24,* 455-476.

McCoy, H.V., Miles, C., & Inciardi, J. (1995). Survival sex: Inner city women and crack cocaine. In J. Inciardi & K. McElrath (Eds.), *The American drug scene* (pp. 172-177). Los Angeles, CA: Roxbury.

Peugh, J. & Belenko, S. (1999). Substance-involved women inmates: Challenges to providing effective treatment. *The Prison Journal, 79*(1), 23-44.

Plasse, B.R. (1995). Parenting groups for recovering addicts in a day treatment center. *Social Work, 40*(1), 65-74.

Prendergast, M.L., Wellisch, J., & Falkin, G.P. (1995). Assessment of and services for substance abusing women offenders in community and correctional settings. *The Prison Journal, 75,* 240-256.

Ramsey, M. (1980). GENESIS: A therapeutic community model for incarcerated female drug offenders. *Contemporary Drug Problems, 93*(3), 273-281.

Regier, D.A., Farmer, M.E., Rae, D.S., Locke, B.Z., Keith, S.J., Judd, L.L., & Goodwin, F.K. (1990). Co-morbidity of mental disorders with alcohol and other drug abuse. *JAMA, 261,* 2511-2518.

Rossi, P.H., Wright, J.D., & Anderson, A.B. (1983). Sample surveys: History, current practice, and future prospects. In P.H. Rossi, J.D. Wright, & A.B. Anderson (Eds.), *Handbook of survey research: Quantitative studies in social relations* (pp. 1-20). New York: Academic Press.

Sanders, J.F., McNeill, K.F., Rienzi, B.M., & DeLouth, T.B. (1997). The incarcerated female felon and substance abuse: Demographics, needs assessment, and program planning for a neglected population. *Journal of Addictions and Offender Counseling, 18*(1), 41-51.

Shearer, R.A. & Baletka, D.M. (1999). Counseling substance abusing offenders: Issues and strategies. *Texas Counseling Association Journal, 27*(2), 71-77.

Shearer, R.A. & Baletka, D.M. (2000). *Female offender—Research and training project.* Huntsville, TX: Correctional Management Institute of Texas.

Sims, B. (2003). The impact of causal attribution on correctional ideology: A national study. *Criminal Justice Review, 28*(1), 1-25.

Szapocznik, J., Kurtines, W.M., Foote, F.H., Perez-Vidal, A., & Hervis, O. (1983). Engaging adolescent drug abusers and their families in treatment: A strategic structured systems approached. *Journal of Consulting and Clinical Psychology, 56,* 552-557.

Teplin, L.A., Abram, K.M., & McClelland, G.M. (1996). Prevalence of psychiatric disorders among incarcerated women. *Archives of General Psychology, 53,* 505-512.

Vigdal, G.L. (1995). *Planning for alcohol and other drug abuse treatment for adults in the criminal justice system: TIP 17.* Rockville, MD: Center for Substance Abuse Treatment, U.S. Department of Health and Human Services.

Wellisch, J., Anglin, M.D., & Prendergast, M. (1993). Numbers and characteristics of drug using women in criminal justice system: Implications for treatment. *Journal of Drug Issues, 23,* 7-30.

Wellisch, J., Prendergast, M.L., & Anglin, M.D. (1994). *Drug abusing women offenders: Results of a national survey.* U.S. Department of Justice, National Institute of Justice.

Wells, D.V.B. & Jackson, J.F. (1992). HIV and chemically dependent women: Recommendations for appropriate health care and drug treatment services. *International Journal of Addiction, 27,* 571-585.

Wilcox, J.A. & Yates, W.R. (1993). Gender and psychiatric co-morbidity in substance abusing individuals. *American Journal on Addictions, 2,* 202-206.

Index

Page numbers followed by the letter "f" indicate figures; those followed by the letter "t" indicate tables.

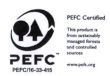

PEFC Certified

This product is
from sustainably
managed forests
and controlled
sources

www.pefc.org

PEFC/16-33-415